Professionalism in Health Care

A Primer for Career Success

3RD EDITION

Sherry Makely, PhD, R.T.(R)
Clarian Health Partners, Inc.
Indianapolis, Indiana

Contributing Author
Vanessa J. Austin, RMA, CAHI
Clarian Health Partners, Inc.
Indianapolis, Indiana

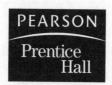
PEARSON

Prentice
Hall

Upper Saddle River, New Jersey 07458

Library of Congress Cataloging-in-Publication Data

Makely, Sherry.
   Professionalism in health care : a primer for career
success / Sherry Makely; contributing author, Vanessa J.
Austin.—3rd ed.
     p. ; cm.
  Includes index.
  ISBN-13: 978-0-13-515387-1
  ISBN-10: 0-13-515387-5
  1. Medical personnel—Professional ethics. 2. Medical
care—Quality control.
  [DNLM: 1. Health Occupations—ethics. 2. Career
Mobility. 3. Ethics, Professional. 4. Interprofessional
Relations. W 21 M235p 2008] I. Austin, Vanessa J. II.
Title.
  R725.5.M35 2008
  610.69—dc22

2007036177

Publisher: Julie Levin Alexander
Publisher's Assistant: Regina Bruno
Executive Editor: Mark Cohen
Associate Editor: Melissa Kerian
Editorial Assistant: Nicole Ragonese
Managing Production Editor: Patrick Walsh
Production Liaison: Cathy O'Connell
Production Editor: Michael Krapovicky,
  Pine Tree Composition
Manufacturing Manager: Ilene Sanford
Manufacturing Buyer: Pat Brown
Art Director: Maria Guglielmo
Cover Designer: Wanda Espana
Director of Marketing: Karen Allman
Marketing Manager: Harper Coles

Marketing Specialist: Michael Sirinides
Media Development Editor: John J. Jordan
New Media Project Manager: Stephen Hartner
Image Resource Center Director: Melinda Patelli
Rights and Permissions Manager: Zina Arabia
Visual Research Manager: Beth Brenzel
Cover Visual Research & Permissions Manager:
  Karen Sanatar
Image Permission Coordinator: Jan Marc
  Quisumbing
Composition: Pine Tree Composition
Printer/Binder: RR Donnelley & Sons
Cover Printer: Phoenix Color Corp./Hagerstown
Cover Photo: Corbis

Pearson Prentice Hall™ is a trademark of Pearson Education, Inc.
Pearson® is a registered trademark of Pearson plc.
Prentice Hall® is a registered trademark of Pearson Education, Inc.

Pearson Education, Ltd., London
Pearson Education Australia Pty. Limited, Sydney
Pearson Education Singapore Pte. Ltd.
Pearson Education North Asia Ltd., Hong Kong
Pearson Education Canada, Ltd., Toronto

Pearson Educación de Mexico, S.A. de C.V.
Pearson Education—Japan, Tokyo
Pearson Education Malaysia, Pte. Ltd.
Pearson Education, Upper Saddle River, New Jersey

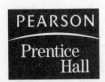

10 9 8 7
ISBN-10: 0-13-515387-5
ISBN-13: 978-0-13-515387-1

Contents

Chapter Five   The Practicum Experience   101
Vanessa J. Austin

Chapter Six   Career Planning and Employment   119

Preface

Who This Book Is for and Why It's Important

Professionalism in Health Care: A Primer for Career Success is designed for students enrolled in nursing and health sciences educational programs in colleges and universities, vocational-technical schools, hospitals, high schools, and on-the-job training programs. This book is also beneficial in orientation sessions for new employees and for in-service and refresher classes for experienced health care workers. Text information is applicable to all health careers and all types, sizes, and locations of health care settings including hospitals, clinics, outpatient facilities, occupational health centers, dental practices, rehabilitation centers, physician practices, surgery centers, home care agencies, mental health facilities, pharmacies, community health centers, nursing homes, transitional and long-term care facilities, satellite imaging and laboratory facilities, public health organizations, urgent care centers, and insurance and billing companies.

This book provides information that is essential to the success of today's health care workers. Hands-on technical skills remain a high priority, but good character, a strong work ethic, and personal and professional traits and behaviors are becoming more important than ever before. Statistics indicate a growing concern with theft, fraud, and behavioral problems in the workplace. Poor attendance, interpersonal conflicts, disregard for quality, and disrespect for authority all too often lead to employees being fired from their jobs. With a growing emphasis on customer service, patient satisfaction, cultural diversity, quality improvement, patient safety, and corporate compliance, health care employers increasingly seek workers with strong "soft skills"—people who communicate appropriately; work well on teams; respect and value differences; use limited resources efficiently; and interact effectively with coworkers, patients, and guests.

Regardless of job title or discipline, every health care student and worker must understand the importance of professionalism and the need to perform in a professional, ethical, legal, and competent manner. Developing and strengthening professional traits and behaviors has become a major challenge for both health care educators and employers. *Professionalism in Health Care: A Primer for Career Success* helps meet that challenge. It describes professional standards that apply to all

vii

health care workers—the "common ground" that everyone shares in providing the highest quality of health care and service excellence for patients, visitors, and guests.

What This Book Covers

Professionalism in Health Care: A Primer for Career Success discusses the following:

- which jobs require professionalism
- definitions and key elements of professionalism
- why professionalism is important to patients, employers, and health care workers
- making a commitment to your job (the "big picture" and where your role fits in, work ethic, attendance, accountability, attitude, quality of work, compliance, representing your employer, and performance evaluation criteria)
- who you are as a person and what you contribute in the workplace (character, values, reputation, integrity, judgment, trustworthiness, honesty, ethics, morals)
- working with others (relationships, teamwork, diversity, respect, manners, communication skills, conflict resolution, customer service)
- how your personal life impacts success on the job (personal image and appearance, personal habits and grammar, professionalism after hours; managing time, personal finances, and stress; problem solving and critical thinking skills; managing change)
- the practicum experience (what to expect during the practicum, internship, externship, or clinical experience and how to ensure success)
- personal and professional growth and advancement (career planning, personal assessments, basic skills, exploring employment opportunities, résumés, interviewing)

Professionalism in Health Care: A Primer for Career Success includes a *Student CD-ROM* in the back of each copy and an *Instructor's Resource Manual* and *Instructor's Resource CD-ROM* that qualified adoptors may request. In addition to chapter readings, the textbook provides a Glossary, What If? Scenarios, Review Questions, and an Appendix containing supplemental samples and material. The companion *Student CD-ROM* presents a series of video scenarios, each demonstrating both professional and unprofessional behaviors. The scenarios feature medical personnel working in a physician practice but the concepts apply to all types of health care workers in a wide variety of settings. The video scenarios correspond with Chapters One through Four and Chapter Six in the textbook and material provided in the *Instructor's Resource Manual* and *Instructor's Resource CD-ROM*. The *Student*

CD-ROM provides learning activities to supplement those listed at the end of each chapter in the textbook. These include Self Assessments with Next Step Improvement Plans, Video Clips and Scenario Analysis Quizzes, Chapter Quizzes, an electronic Résumé Builder, and additional Learning Opportunities linked to each chapter in the textbook.

Information for Students

Students should read each chapter in the textbook and complete the end-of-chapter learning activities before proceeding to the next chapter. Text end-of-chapter learning activities include What If? Scenarios and Review Questions. Students should also complete *Student CD-ROM* activities including the Scenario Analysis Quizzes, Self Assessments and Next Step Improvement Plans, Chapter Quizzes, Learning Opportunities, and other chapter-specific assignments.

Information for Instructors

The *Instructor's Resource Manual* and *Instructor's Resource CD-ROM* provide print and electronic course material that offers versatility in structuring student learning experiences. Material is ideal for traditional classroom courses and can also be electronically downloaded onto an on-line learning environment for both instructor-facilitated as well as independent study courses. *Professionalism in Health Care: A Primer for Career Success* may be used as:

1. textbook for a classroom-based, instructor-led course (using the *Student CD-ROM, Instructor's Resource Manual* and *Instructor's Resource CD-ROM*)
2. textbook for an instructor-facilitated on-line or independent study course (a self-paced, learn-on-your-own approach using the *Student CD-ROM* and the *Independent Study Guide* provided in the *Instructor's Resource Manual*)
3. personal reading for self-instruction and review.

The *Instructor's Resource Manual* provides:

- guidelines for using material for classroom, on-line, and self-study courses
- details for using PowerPoint slides, dress code photographs, samples, and other material on the *Instructor's Resource CD-ROM*
- template for an easily modified, six-chapter lesson plan
- course description and course objectives
- questions with answers mapped to chapter objectives and text material.

The *Instructor's Resource Manual* also includes the following for each chapter of the course:

- objectives and curriculum outline
- lesson plan with discussion topics and recommended learning experiences
- answers to Review Questions
- essay answers to text What If? Scenarios, plus multiple choice options and answers
- answers to *Student CD-ROM* Chapter Quizzes and Scenario Analysis Quizzes

The *Instructor's Resource Manual* also provides an Independent Study Guide to assist in developing on-line and independent study courses. Used in conjunction with the textbook and *Student CD-ROM*, the Independent Study Guide provides a self-paced or structured approach as determined by the facilitator.

The Instructor's Resource CD-ROM provides:

- an electronic version of the *Instructor's Resource Manual*
- glossary from the text
- an electronic test generator for customized pre/post chapter tests and comprehensive final exams
- PowerPoint slides for classroom lectures
- photographic examples of compliance and non-compliance with professional dress code standards
- a sample job description, performance evaluation, job application form, résumé, résumé cover letter, and interview follow-up letter from the Appendix in the text
- pertinent material from the Student CD-ROM.

Electronic course material can be down loaded onto an on-line learning environment. Downloadable content includes video clips and other material from the *Student CD-ROM* as well as the electronic TestGen questions, PowerPoint slides, and PDF files from the *Instructor's Resource CD-ROM*. The *Instructor's Resource Manual* is provided in editable Microsoft Word format on the *Instructor's Resource CD-ROM*. With the exception of PDF files, all material on the *Instructor's Resource CD-ROM* may be edited by the instructor. Prentice Hall provides technical downloading assistance for on-line course applications.

Professionalism in Health Care: A Primer for Career Success is designed for all types of nursing and health sciences students enrolled in college and university programs, vocational-technical programs, hospital-based programs, high school health occupations programs, and on-the-job training programs.

The textbook and *Student CD-ROM* materials may be incorporated into introductory, core curriculum, and capstone courses in nursing or health sciences, Professionalism, Medical Law and Ethics, or Office Management and Business. Additionally, this text can be used as preparation for an internship/externship/practicum or in classes or seminars on topics such as Employment Strategies, Career Development, and Work Readiness. Instructors may wish to use this text in general introductory courses and then supplement the students' learning later on in a more advanced, discipline-specific course.

The textbook and *Student CD-ROM* may also be used in orientation sessions for new employees or for in-service or refresher courses for experienced health care workers to:

- describe professional performance expectations
- emphasize customer service and standards of care behaviors
- reinforce corporate mission, values, teamwork, and quality improvement initiatives
- outline corporate compliance, HIPAA, and policy/procedure training
- support performance improvement, skills enhancement, and career planning activities.

In Closing

We hope you find *Professionalism in Health Care: A Primer for Career Success* and its companion materials informative, thought provoking, and beneficial.

Reviewers

Jean Beckner, BSRS, RDMS, RVT
Assistant Professor, Diagnostic Medical
Sonography
Cuyahoga Community College
Parma, Ohio

Norma Bird, M.Ed., BS, CMA
Program Director, Medical Assisting
Idaho State University
Pocatello, Idaho

Robert Freeland, MBA
Professor, Business and Health Care
Administration
Columbia Southern University
Orange Beach, Alabama

Robert Garrie, MPA, RHIA
Assistant Professor, Health Information
Management
Alabama State University
Montgomery, Alabama

Denise Grant, RN, MSN, CMA
Assistant Dean of Health Sciences
Northwestern Technical College
Rock Springs, Georgia

Charlotte A. Jensen, BS, MPA/HAS, CMA
Program Chair, Medical Assisting
Cabrillo College
Aptos, California

Katherine B. Lee, CST, MS
Professor, Surgical Technology
Richland Community College
Decatur, Illinois

Julie Pepper, CMA, BS
Instructor, Medical Assisting
Chippewa Valley Technical College
Eau Claire, Wisconsin

Alisa Petree, MHSM, MT(ASCP)
Instructor/Clinical Coordinator, Medical
Laboratory Technician
McLennan Community College
Waco, Texas

Amy Schultz, RN, BSN, MS
Program Director for Non-Credit Health
Careers
Angelina College
Lufkin, Texas

Shawna Strickland, MEd, RRT-NPS, AE-C
Assistant Professor/Director of Clinical
Education, Respiratory Therapy
University of Missouri – Columbia
Columbia, Missouri

Cheryl Vineyard, CMA, CPC
Program Director, Medical Assisting
Eastern New Mexico University
Roswell, New Mexico

Special thanks to the following health care professionals for their assistance with the "Unique Professionalism Challenges" section in Chapter Four:

Sherri Alexander, CST
Lula Atkins, D.T.R.
Linda Courtier, RN
Debby Ferguson, M.S., REEG/RPT, RPSGT, RNCST
Jesse Fleming
Lynn Fulk, B.S., CNMT, FSNMTS, ARRT(R)
Deborah Grider, CPC-EMS, CPC-H, CPC-P, CCS-P, RMC
Debra Hampton, LPN, BSPH, CPC, CCS-P
Lindi Holt, Ph.D., NREMT-P, ATC
Fran Klene, B.S., M.S., RDMS/RT-retired
Oliver, Cheryl, M.S., MT(ASCP)
Donna Thaler Long, MSM, RT(R)(M)(QM)
J.A. Mishler, D.D.S.
Mary Mohr, RPh, M.S.
Mary Rehmel, LDH, B.S.
Dan R. Strahan, B.S. RT(T) ARRT
Linda VanScoder, Ed.D., RRT

Special thanks to Carmen Martin (photographer), Terry Brooks-Allen and Damon Hynds (models), and the following Clarian Health Medical Assisting faculty and students for their assistance with the dress code photography:

Marsha Wilson, BS, Program Director
Vanessa Austin, RMA, CAHI, Clinical Coordinator
Student models:
Kelley Beagle
Iesha Dinwiddie
Rustyna Hodo
Madonna Key
Debbie Landrey
Kimberly Milstead
Dinh Sizemore
Sara Unthank

Health Care Professionals

Recognition as a health care professional is something that has to be earned—a reputation that's developed and maintained each and every day you come to work. Professionalism is a state of mind, a way of "being," "knowing," and "doing" that sets you apart from others. It gives direction to how you look, behave, think, and act. It brings together who you are as a person, what you value, how you treat other people, what you contribute in the workplace, and how seriously you take your job. Professionals don't just work to earn a paycheck. Income is important, but professionals view their work as a source of pride and a reflection of the role they play in society.

Health care professionals are good at what they do—and they like doing it. They enjoy helping others and knowing they've made a difference. Professionals have their "act together"—and it shows. They set high standards for their performance and achieve them. They see the "big picture" in health care and know where they fit in. Professionals care about quality and how to improve it. They treat everyone they meet with dignity and respect. And they continually strive to grow and to learn.

Introduction

Opportunity is missed by most because it is dressed in overalls and looks like work.

Thomas Alva Edison, Inventor, 1847–1931

Recognition as a Health Care Professional

There's no doubt about it. When you're sick or injured, or when a family member or friend needs health care, you want to be certain that you and your loved ones are cared for by professionals. Thinking back to the times when you've had a doctor's appointment, visited an outpatient clinic or emergency room, or been hospitalized for tests or treatments, you probably encountered many different types of health care workers. Although most of these workers performed their duties in a professional manner, you may have encountered a few who did not. We would like to think that everyone who works in health care functions as a professional, but experience has shown that such is not always the case.

What is a professional? How can you recognize a professional when you see one? What does "taking a professional approach" to one's work mean? Why is professionalism important? What must you learn as a student to prepare you for future recognition as a health care professional yourself?

According to *Webster's New World Dictionary of the American Language, College Edition*, a *professional* is a person "with much experience and great skill in a specified role" who is "engaged in a specific occupation for pay or as a means of livelihood." As we look around us, we see many examples of professionals in different walks of life. In sports, for example, professional status is awarded to gifted athletes who have surpassed amateur events and moved into high-paying, major league competitions. In medicine, law, and science, people like doctors, lawyers, and engineers are considered professionals because of their expertise, college education, and special credentials such as licenses and certifications. But truck drivers, hair stylists, and photographers consider themselves as professionals too, as do bankers, insurance underwriters, and investment counselors. Exactly what is a professional and who is qualified to be one?

Occupations are sometimes divided into "professional" and "nonprofessional" categories based on criteria such as:

- unique and exclusive scopes of practice
- minimum educational standards and accreditation of educational programs
- minimum standards for entry into practice
- required credentials such as licenses or certifications
- professional associations with codes of ethics and competency standards.

When we apply these criteria to the health care workforce, doctors, registered nurses, pharmacists, physical therapists, medical assistants, surgical technologists, dental assistants, radiographers, and the like are all classified as professionals. That leaves all the other types of people who work for health care organizations in the non-professional classification, including secretaries, insurance claims processors, food service workers, environmental services and maintenance personnel, admitting clerks, telephone operators, landscaping and grounds personnel, equipment repair technicians, laboratory assistants, and scores of other employees. Not making the list of "professionals" can be demeaning to people who work hard and make their jobs a top priority in their lives. So in health care it's important to acknowledge another set of criteria that give every type of worker the opportunity to be regarded as a "professional." Regardless of how other people may classify your job as "professional" or "nonprofessional," it's what you contribute in the workplace that really matters. *What* you do and *how* you do it are extremely important, whether you provide hands-on care or function in a support role behind the scenes. In fact, in the everyday life of health care organizations throughout the country, it's much more important to differentiate between *professionals* and *unprofessionals*.

Everyone who provides direct patient care or who works in a supportive role is eligible for, and should strive for, recognition as a professional. Professional recognition isn't something that's automatically bestowed upon a person when he or she completes an educational program, obtains a degree or certificate, or secures a license to practice. It's not dependent on a person's socioeconomic status, income, age, gender, race, job title, or position within the hierarchy of an organization. After all, we've all known people with college degrees, special credentials, and impressive job titles who don't behave in a professional manner.

Recognition as a health care professional is something that has to be earned—a reputation that's developed and maintained each and every day you come to work. Professionalism is a state of mind, a way of "being," "knowing," and "doing" that sets you apart from others. It gives direction to how you look, behave, think, and act. It brings together who you are as a person, what you value, how you treat other people, what you contribute in the workplace, and how seriously you take your job. Professionals don't just work to earn a paycheck. Income is important, but professionals view their work as a source of pride and a reflection of the role they play in society.

If you're serious about a career in health care, viewing yourself as a professional and being recognized as such by other people will be a major key to your success. Professionalism is something every organization looks for in its employees. How can you spot a health care professional when you see one? It's easy.

Health care professionals are good at what they do—and they like doing it. They enjoy helping others and knowing they've made a difference. Professionals have their "act together"—and it shows. They set high standards for their performance and achieve them. They see the "big picture" in health care and know where they fit in. Professionals care about quality and how to improve it. They treat everyone they meet with dignity and respect. And they continually strive to grow and to learn.

Spotting a health care professional may be easy—but becoming one yourself is another matter. It's something you have to concentrate on every day—but it's worth it. To *be* a professional, you must *feel like* a professional. In our society, the amount of education a person has and what he or she does for a living have become important contributors to an individual's self-esteem and sense of self-worth. *What we do* has become *who we are*. When you graduate from an educational program, earn a degree, or obtain a license or certification you experience the exhilaration of knowing you've accomplished something worthwhile. Being recognized by others as a professional brings value and meaning to your efforts. It reminds you that what you do counts. This is true whether you care for patients, process specimens, coordinate paperwork, prepare meals, clean public areas, order and stock supplies, or work in any one of a hundred different health care jobs. It's also true whether you work in a hospital, physician/dental practice, clinic, long-term care facility, or some other type of health care organization. No matter what your role involves, how you view your work and how you approach it can have a tremendous impact on your own life as well as on the lives of those you serve.

Why Health Care Needs Professionals

Health care is a basic need for survival. Each year, millions of Americans receive health services in doctor's offices, hospitals, dental practices, outpatient clinics, mental health facilities, and in their homes. Patients rely on health care professionals to provide affordable, state-of-the-art diagnostic and therapeutic procedures to help them overcome illness, injury, and other abnormalities that impact their health and quality of life.

But health care is a business too and as consumers and taxpayers, we all pay for health services. Finding new ways to provide services for more patients, using fewer resources, while achieving higher quality outcomes has become a major challenge for health care providers. The only way this challenge can be met is through a cadre of well-qualified employees committed to quality and cost effectiveness. People who fail to take a professional approach to their work are often absent, late, unreliable, and sloppy. Their actions may endanger quality of care, customer service, safety, and the efficient use of limited resources.

Working in health care requires special skills and an attitude that supports service to others. Patients seek health care services during some of the most vulnerable times in their lives, when they're sick, injured, and "at their worst." Each patient–worker interaction must build confidence and trust. The decisions and actions of those who care for patients, or those who work behind the scenes to support the efforts of caregivers, can have an immediate and lasting impact.

The Importance of Every Job and Every Worker

No matter what job you will have, you will play an important role in health care. No job is insignificant and no worker is unimportant. Let's face reality—if a job wasn't important it wouldn't exist. Your challenge is to pull together the mixture of knowledge, skills, compassion, and commitment required to make you the very best employee you can possibly be. If you can meet this challenge and carry it through on a daily basis, then you've earned the privilege of being recognized as a health care professional. Nothing less is acceptable.

Professionalism in Health Care: A Primer for Career Success can help you on your journey toward professional recognition. The basic elements of professionalism are discussed, along with the personal and professional characteristics and behaviors that you need to be successful in your career.

Every health care employee has the opportunity and the obligation to strive for professional recognition. Always remember—it's not *the job you do* that makes you a professional, it's *how you do it* that counts.

It's important to start down the road to professionalism while still a student. If your educational program includes a practicum requirement (i.e., internship, externship, or clinical observations or rotations), you will be interacting with health care workers, physicians, patients, visitors, and guests to gain hands-on experience before you graduate. Chapter Five will help you prepare for success in your practicum. Even if your program does not include a practicum requirement, you will still find the information presented in Chapter Five informative and insightful when starting your new job upon graduation.

There are several things you can do now as a student to support your quest for eventual recognition as a health care professional. Apply yourself, take your studies seriously, learn how to manage your time, and hone your communication skills. Make good decisions, look out for your fellow classmates, and find ways to balance the competing priorities in your life. Everything that you hear, observe, learn, and experience will be important at some point in your health career. Expect some changes along the way and plan to continue learning and growing well after you've completed your initial education. Most important, always strive to do your very best. You and the patients you will some day serve deserve nothing less.

chapter one

Making a Commitment to Your Job

"I'm a great believer in luck and I find the harder I work, the more I have of it."

Thomas Jefferson, 3rd U.S. President, 1743–1826

"A pessimist sees the difficulty in every opportunity. An optimist sees the opportunity in every difficulty."

Winston Churchill, British Prime Minister, 1874–1965

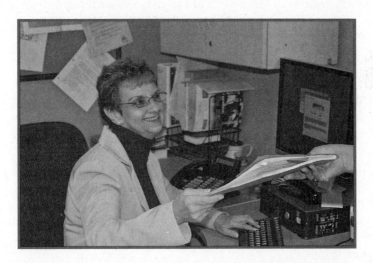

Professionalism in Action

The Student CD-ROM that accompanies this book contains video scenarios and other learning activities related to this chapter. Once you complete reading this chapter, turn to the CD-ROM to gain a richer understanding of the concepts presented here.

Chapter Objectives

Having completed this chapter, you will be able to:

- Identify three factors that positively impact recognition as a health care professional.
- List eight health care jobs that are important and require professionalism.
- Explain the importance of a systems perspective.
- Identify five factors that demonstrate a strong work ethic.
- Differentiate between the terms *accountable, reliable,* and *diligent.*
- Describe the attitudinal differences between optimists and pessimists.
- Define *corporate compliance, conflict of interest*, and *whistle blower*.
- Discuss the importance of confidentiality and HIPAA.
- Identify how competence and scope of practice impact quality of care.
- Define *corrective action* and list five behaviors that could result in job dismissal.
- Explain the purpose of performance evaluations and list three ways to prepare for one.
- Differentiate between objective and subjective evaluation criteria.

Key Terms

360-degree feedback
accountable
caregivers
certification
competence
confidentiality
conflict of interest
contingency plans
corporate compliance
corporate mission
corporate values
corrective action
diligent
discretion
dismissal
front-line workers
goals
hierarchy
HIPAA

hostile workplace
impaired
insubordination
license
objective
optimists
organizational chart
peers
performance evaluations
perspective
pessimists
probationary period
punctual
reliable
scope of practice
sexual harassment
stagnant
subjective
subordinates

systems perspective   vendors
traits   work ethic
unethical   whistle blower

The Jobs that Require Professionalism

As discussed in the Introduction, no job is insignificant and no worker is unimportant. Just think about it. Everyone knows the roles of doctors, nurses, pharmacists, and physical therapists, for example, are important. But patients and the general public may not be as familiar with the roles of other **caregivers** such as medical assistants, radiographers, EKG technicians, nuclear medicine technologists, occupational therapists, and sonographers, just to name a few. People who work in support roles, often behind the scenes, may be even less known to patients and the general public. This includes billing clerks, instrument technicians, biomedical engineers, financial analysts, research assistants, and the scores of other kinds of personnel whose roles are also vital in health care. Depending on how you add them up, there are several hundred different jobs in health care organizations. Large urban hospitals and medical centers employ so many different types of workers, they begin to resemble small towns.

If your job will involve direct patient care, it should be obvious that professionalism is important. The same holds true with jobs where workers interact with visitors, guests, and vendors. Examples include customer service agents, telephone operators, purchasing agents, accounts payable clerks, insurance processors, and departmental secretaries. But what about the large percentage of health care workers who work in support roles behind the scenes? If they don't interact directly with patients, visitors, guests, or **vendors,** is professionalism really important in their jobs, too? Let's take a closer look.

What if environmental services workers (housekeepers) neglected to empty trash containers in public rest rooms for several days, miscalculated the dilution of an antiseptic cleaning fluid, or used the wrong wax on the floor of a busy hallway? What if food service workers put the wrong items on a special-diet patient tray, neglected to wash their hands after a trip to the rest room, or spilled hot grease near an open flame in the kitchen? What if central service technicians packaged the wrong supplies, failed to replace outdated stock, or operated sterilizers at the wrong temperature?

It should be obvious that professionalism is vital in every job. Each job exists for a reason. If there weren't a need for a job and having the responsibilities of that job performed appropriately, the job wouldn't exist. So it only stands to reason that every job is important—and doing the job well requires a professional approach to one's work.

The Big Picture and Where You Fit In

No matter what your eventual job may entail, perspective is important. You must be able to step back and view "the big picture" to see where your role fits in. As a health care worker, you will be part of one of the nation's largest and fastest growing industries. How much do you know about the industry in which you work? Are you up-to-speed on the latest trends and issues in health care? Do you have a national perspective on America's health care system—its history, current status, and where it seems to be headed? Do you know enough about the health care scene in your own part of the country to discuss how local issues compare with national trends?

Because you work in health care, other people who don't may look to you for information or advice. Because we are all consumers and taxpaying supporters of health care, most everyone has an opinion to share or a concern to discuss. People may ask you questions such as:

"What is managed care?"

"What is an HMO?"

"Why can't I go to any doctor I want to anymore?"

"What is a primary care physician?"

"Why are the two hospitals in town merging together?"

"Why did our hospital let some of its staff go?"

"Where are the best job and career opportunities in health care?"

Can you answer questions like these? If you want to be viewed as a professional, you need to be aware of what's going on in your industry and be able to talk intelligently about it with other people. This doesn't mean that you have to be a walking encyclopedia on health care. But you should keep up with the latest trends and issues on both the local and national levels. Be on the lookout for information from a variety of sources. Read articles about health care in newspapers and magazines. Watch the news on television and look for special programs about health care. Attend seminars on health care topics whenever you get the opportunity. Become active in a professional association. Talk with people who are current on the latest information and join in conversations to learn more yourself and to share what you already know with others.

Equally important to having an awareness of the big picture is knowing where you will fit into that picture—especially within the organization where you will work. This begins by developing a **systems perspective**—standing back, viewing the entire process of how a patient moves through the organization, and seeing how your job fits into that process. No one in health care works in a vacuum. That is, everyone's work is interconnected. Only when your efforts are well coordinated with those of other employees can your company conduct its business and fulfill its mission.

Think about the job for which you are preparing and the responsibilities you will have. How will your responsibilities connect with those of other workers? How will your role interact with the roles of other workers to fulfill the company's mission? What other workers will you have to depend on to get your work done? What other workers will have to depend on you to get their work done? Where do the patients fit into this continuum of efforts? What must you do to comply with HIPAA and other laws to protect the rights of patients and ensure high quality health care? Most companies have an **organizational chart**—an illustration showing the components of the company and how they fit together. Typical organizational charts include the **hierarchy** of the company—people and work units that are arranged by rank. In other words, "who" reports "to whom." Large companies have detailed illustrations showing the flow of work processes across and among different departments. Regardless of the company and its structure, there is one common thread—all departments and all employees must depend on each other to get the work done and done well.

From a systems perspective, ask yourself the question, "What could happen if I don't take a professional approach to my work and get things done in an appropriate manner?" What if you fail to show up for work without notifying someone or arrive several minutes or hours late for your shift? What if you "drop the ball" and don't follow through on an assignment or job duty? What if you get sloppy and make a mistake? What if you aren't concentrating on what you are doing and miss something important? What if you show up for work **impaired** by alcohol or some other drug? What if you ignore policies or violate **confidentiality?** What if you let your skills slip and don't keep up on a new procedure or piece of equipment? What effect will an "I don't care" attitude have on your job performance?

What impact will your performance have on the organization for which you work and on the patients it serves? Remember, if your job weren't important, it would not exist. So just how important is it? Professionals can answer that question easily because they see the big picture and they know exactly where they fit in. They know that other people are counting on them and they can predict what might happen if they don't follow through.

If you don't perform your job well by meeting the expectations that management has set forth for your position, you won't be in that job for very long. You may be able to hide incompetence, sloppiness, and indifference for a little while, but eventually poor performance will catch up with you. What's worse, someone (or several people) could be victimized by your lack of professionalism in the meantime. If any of these "what ifs" sound like they might apply to you and how you approach your work, make a conscious decision right now to change your ways and improve—and keep reading.

A Strong Work Ethic

Ask any employer what characteristic is most important in a good employee and the majority will respond, "A strong **work ethic.**" This means positioning your job as a high priority in your life and making sound decisions about how you approach your work. Employees with a strong work ethic stay focused and leave their personal problems at home. They apply themselves to the task at hand and take a thorough approach to getting the work done right—the first time. They exercise self-discipline and self-control. They know what management expects of them and they measure up. They don't wait to be told what to do and they demonstrate a positive attitude and enthusiasm for their work.

Let's examine some of the factors involved in developing a strong work ethic and demonstrating a commitment to your job and to the organization that employs you.

Attendance and Punctuality

It's nearly impossible to demonstrate a commitment to your job without being there. Performing the duties of your job requires showing up for work every day and being **punctual.**

Poor attendance usually results in other people having to cover for you when you aren't there yourself. How does it make you feel when your coworkers call in sick frequently, leaving you to do your work plus theirs? How do you think they feel when your attendance leaves a lot to be desired? Many health care organizations are already lean on staffing and can't afford to have people absent on a regular basis. It's important to be there when people are counting on you—and to arrive on time.

When you arrive late for work, you hold things up and inconvenience other people. A patient's procedure might have to be rescheduled, possibly delaying someone's diagnosis, treatment, surgery, or discharge from the hospital. Needed supplies might not get delivered on time, paperwork might be filed too late to meet a deadline, or other people might have to work beyond their shifts to get caught up. Remember how the roles of health care workers are interconnected? You may think that arriving late for your own job is not a problem, but what kinds of complications are you causing other people?

Most everyone must miss work or arrive late on occasion. But when poor attendance or punctuality becomes a habit, it also becomes a performance issue and possible grounds for **corrective action** (steps taken to overcome a job performance problem) or **dismissal.**

Make a commitment to show up for work every day, arrive on time, and be ready to work when your shift starts. Have **contingency plans** to cover situations when your children or spouse gets sick or when your transportation is unreliable. Protect your health and safety to keep from getting sick or injured yourself. Eat well, make sure you get enough sleep, think about getting a flu shot, and avoid unnecessary risks that might injure you.

When you arrive at work, give yourself enough time to park your car or get from the bus stop to your work area a few minutes early. When your shift starts, be sure you're in the area and ready to go. It's always better to arrive a little early than a little late. Supervisors notice who shows up early and who's in place, ready to work when the shift begins.

Don't take excessively long or unscheduled breaks. Try to allow some extra time at the end of your shift in case you get held over. Never leave a patient, coworker, visitor, or guest "hanging" by rushing out the door the minute your shift ends. It's your responsibility to stay long enough to complete your work or to hand it off to the person who follows you. Make sure there's a smooth transition between shifts and don't leave your work for other people to finish up. As mentioned previously, your job is important or it wouldn't exist. People are counting on you to get your part of the work done.

Reliability and Accountability

Being **reliable** and **accountable** are key factors in professionalism. If someone agrees to help you and then doesn't follow through, how does that make you feel? If getting your work done on time depends on other people getting their work done on time, what happens when someone drops the ball? From a systems perspective, each worker is responsible for completing the duties of his or her job appropriately so that other people can complete their work, too. Make sure you get your own work done on time so you don't hold other people up. If you've told someone he or she can count on you, prove you are a reliable person and follow through. If you're there for others when you say you will be, it's more likely that other people will be there for you when you need them. Following through on commitments is a big part of the team effort.

Accepting responsibility and the consequences of your actions is also important. Professionals hold themselves personally accountable and avoid shifting the blame to others. If you make a mistake (and everyone does occasionally), admit it and accept full responsibility. Apologize to those who have been inconvenienced and remember—although it's important to apologize for a mistake, the apology does not erase the fact that a mistake was made. Learn from the experience and avoid making the same mistake twice. Your supervisor, coworkers, and other people will appreciate your "the buck stops here" attitude.

Accept all work assignments for which you are qualified and prepared to perform. If you are given a work assignment that you are not qualified or prepared to perform, discuss the situation with your supervisor immediately. Refusal to complete a task as assigned may be construed as **insubordination** and grounds for dismissal. Yet a responsible person would never perform a task that he or she is not capable of performing appropriately. When serving the needs of patients, it's important to avoid passing judgment or projecting your own personal beliefs on others. If you object to an assignment because it conflicts with your religious beliefs, morals, or values, you must discuss these concerns with your supervisor. It's best to resolve issues like these when you first consider a job offer. If you wish to not participate in abortions, sex change operations, end-of-life procedures, or other such activities, many employers will allow you to opt out, but this must be discussed ahead of time so patient care is not delayed or jeopardized.

Attitude and Enthusiasm

How often have you witnessed another person's behavior and thought to yourself, "What a negative attitude!" For some people, a negative attitude is a way of life. As **pessimists,** they see the glass as half empty. From their perspective, their situation is always bad and getting worse. They complain about everything and nothing seems to satisfy them. They rarely smile, appear happy, or convey enthusiasm about their work. They can spread negativity to everyone around them and undermine morale, teamwork, and a spirit of cooperation.

Optimists, on the other hand, display a positive attitude most of the time. They see the glass as half full and approach life with enthusiasm. When they experience things they don't like, they voice their complaints in a constructive manner. They look for reasons to feel happy and content and they appreciate the small things in life. They tend to smile a lot and convey a friendly and cooperative attitude.

Are you an optimist or a pessimist? How does your approach to life affect your work and your relationships with other people? When you confront a situation, do you automatically look for the good in it, or the bad? Do you focus on the positives of the situation or the negatives? Two different people may look at the same situation in two very different ways. It's all a matter of **perspective.** Here's an example. Your department is implementing a new computer software program to automate the tracking of patient records. The software must be customized to your facility and then tested to make sure it works accurately. During the development and testing stages, you and your coworkers must enter and retrieve patient records using both the old and the new systems. This transitional phase results in more work and requires additional training, participation in committee meetings, and written forms to complete. How would you react? What attitude would you display? Would you become negative and complain about the extra work and how unfairly you are being treated? Or would you take the positive approach and accept the extra work, knowing the new system will eventually make things better? Your choice is clear. You can focus on the negatives, whine about your immediate circumstances, and make your life, and the lives of those around you, miserable. Or, you can focus on the positives, think about the future when things will get better, and support a spirit of teamwork and cooperation. How would you want your coworkers to react to this same situation?

Displaying enthusiasm and a positive attitude is an important part of a professional's work ethic. If you expect to excel in your work and advance in your career, you must have a positive attitude. If you're an optimist, make sure your positive attitude is evident at work. If you tend towards being a pessimist, you can change your outlook if you wish to but doing so will take some effort on your part. Start looking for the bright side in any situation and focus on the positives. Seize opportunities to feel happy and develop an appreciation for the small things in life. When you must complain, express your concerns in a constructive manner. If you feel "stressed out" or experience the early stages of "burn out," get some help right away. Health care workers who don't alleviate their stress run the risk of transferring negativism to coworkers and patients. Too many professionals "burn out" early in their careers due to negative, unpleasant work environments created by coworkers who failed to resolve their stress. Smile every chance you get, even when speaking on the telephone. By adopting a positive attitude, you will experience more joy and greater satisfaction in life, and your optimism and enthusiasm will spread to those around you.

Quality of Work

No matter where your job falls within the organizational structure of your company, the quality of your work is extremely important. What does quality mean to you? What do you think quality means to the company who will employ you? What does quality mean to the patients you will serve? Think about how your efforts support quality. What factors can you identify that erode quality?

Quality requires **competence**—possessing the necessary knowledge and skills to perform your job appropriately and safely on a daily basis. Make sure you are well trained and competent to perform each and every function associated with your job. Never take a chance and just "wing" it. Although your supervisor will probably evaluate your competence and review your work performance periodically, it's up to you to keep your knowledge up-to-date and your skills sharp. Learn about the latest procedures, techniques, and new equipment. Attend in-service sessions and continuing education workshops and read publications in your field. Never hesitate to ask questions or request help. And remember, just because you've completed your training doesn't mean your education ends. Nothing stays **stagnant** in health care. You must always keep learning and striving for ways to improve the quality of your work. As a professional, it's your responsibility.

Perhaps you've heard the saying "Quality is in the details." This means making even the smallest error or overlooking even the most minute detail can have a negative impact on quality. This includes putting stock items on the wrong shelf, misfiling a patient's record, losing a telephone number, miscalculating a bill, forgetting to order next week's supplies, or missing an important meeting because you forgot to write it down. Each day there are thousands of opportunities for details to fall through the cracks. Being **diligent** about quality can help prevent these kinds of problems.

Taking an unprofessional approach to your work can certainly damage quality. Being lazy or sloppy, not paying attention, working while impaired, operating equipment without proper training, or ignoring safety precautions can all lead to serious outcomes. You could hurt yourself or someone else, damage expensive equipment, waste valuable resources, or put yourself and your employer legally at risk. Make sure you pay attention to what you are doing, work in a safe and conscientious manner, and always look for opportunities to improve the quality of your work.

It's also important to contribute to quality improvement company-wide. No one has a better handle on how to improve work processes and quality outcomes than the people who actually do the work on a daily basis. Management can't improve the company's quality without the help of **subordinates.** When you have a suggestion for quality improvement, submit it to your supervisor. When you spot a potential problem area, report it. If your area or department receives periodic quality-related data, pay attention to the reports and do your best to help make improvements.

Responding to a request by stating, "That's not my job!" is unacceptable. Doing what's asked of you might not fall within your job duties, but one of two things needs to happen. Either you should go ahead and perform the task because you're capable of doing it and willing or you should refer the matter to the appropriate person and then make sure he or she follows through. No task is too menial when working in health care. If a patient or visitor becomes ill in the parking garage, stay there and offer assistance or send for help. If someone looks lost, ask if you can provide directions. If you notice a spill in a public hallway, don't wait for a housekeeper to discover it. Either clean it up yourself (using safety precautions) or report it to the appropriate person and then remain in the area until it's cleaned up to prevent any unnecessary injuries. If you observe that a piece of equipment is not working properly or spot a situation that might pose a health or safety hazard to someone else, don't just go on about your business. Take action! A commitment to quality means paying attention to what's going on around you and addressing concerns before they escalate into serious problems.

Evaluating Performance

A commitment to quality, good attendance, and a positive attitude are all components of a strong work ethic. Employers will monitor your work ethic and evaluate your performance on a regular basis. Let's take a look at how your on-the-job performance will be evaluated so that you can keep this process in mind as you continue your reading.

Unlike passing a final exam and then moving on to the next course, the "demonstration of mastery" on the job is ongoing each and every day. If you lack the competence, interpersonal skills, or commitment required to perform your job effectively, your deficiencies will soon become apparent. If, however, you take your job seriously and practice what you are learning in this text, you should be well prepared for exemplary job performance.

The terminology and processes used to conduct **performance evaluations** vary from company to company. Sometimes the evaluation tools are called "performance appraisals" and the overall evaluation process is called "performance management." The purpose of performance evaluations is not to determine how well the employee is "liked" or how his/her supervisor "feels" about the employee (i.e., **subjective** criteria). Instead, employers seek to evaluate job performance using **objective** criteria based on competence, behaviors (i.e., customer service, teamwork, problem solving), and **traits** (i.e., attitude, appearance, initiative). Employers attempt to evaluate traits such as "appearance" and "attitude" because they are so important to job performance. But traits such as these are difficult to measure objectively. It's almost impossible to remove all subjectivity from the evaluation process. Performance may be evaluated using two sets of behavioral criteria. One set of behaviors is expected of all employees, with a second set that applies only to workers in certain job classifications.

It's not unusual for new employees to undergo a **probationary period** whereby their attendance and performance are closely monitored to make sure the employee is a "good fit" for the organization and the position. The employee is evaluated at the end of his/her probationary period and the decision is made to retain the employee or not. Having successfully completed their probationary period, employees are then subject to regular performance evaluations from that point forward, typically on an annual basis.

Small organizations may evaluate employee performance on an informal basis. The supervisor observes the employee's performance over a period of time and then provides oral feedback regarding strengths, weaknesses, and areas for improvement. This "oral feedback evaluation" may or may not be documented in writing and maintained as part of the employee's personnel file. Larger companies typically evaluate employee performance on a more formal basis. The supervisor observes the employee's performance during the year, completes a written performance evaluation form at the designated time, and meets with the employee to discuss the results. The performance evaluation form and follow-up meeting are documented in writing and maintained in the employee's personnel file. (Refer to the Appendix for a sample performance evaluation.) An increasing number of employers now use **360-degree feedback** evaluation methods. To obtain 360-degree feedback, input is solicited from several people who have worked with the employee being evaluated, not just from his/her supervisor. This may include **peers**, subordinates, team members, customers, people from other departments, and people outside the organization. Having input from more people helps reduce subjectivity and provides a broader view of the employee's performance. For employees who work on teams, soliciting feedback from team members helps evaluate the employee's "team work" and extends the evaluation beyond just individual performance.

The performance evaluation process not only captures information about the previous year, it also lays out plans for the coming year. Through discussions with supervisors, employees develop **goals,** well-defined stepping-stones that help you progress from where you are now to where you eventually want to be. They identify methods to overcome deficiencies, enhance skills, and work towards job advancement. The majority of employees will likely receive "average" evaluations. Employees who receive "poor" evaluations are put "on notice" that improvements are expected or termination may result. Employees who receive "excellent" evaluations may be slotted for promotional opportunities. Which behaviors result in "excellent" evaluations? Keep reading this text! Most everything you need to know in order to earn an excellent evaluation is contained in these chapters. Pay attention to the "Next Step Improvement Plans" presented for each chapter on your Student CD-ROM. Evaluate your own strengths and weaknesses and begin developing your plans for improvement. Learn as much as you can from the assessments and other types of evaluations you undergo while still a student. Each day you acquire more knowledge and experience to improve your performance. Keep in mind—performance evaluations conducted by employers don't just result in feedback about how well you're doing. More and more companies are now tying the amount of an individual's annual pay increase to his/her performance evaluation score. Employees who receive high scores on their performance evaluations receive higher pay raises than employees who receive low scores. Employees who score below acceptable levels likely receive no pay raise and face termination unless improvements are made.

Regardless of your company's policies and procedures, a performance evaluation is an excellent way to get feedback on how well your supervisor thinks you function in your job and what you can do to increase your value to the organization. Don't wait until a few days before your review to prepare—prepare all year long. Make sure you have a copy of your job description. Job descriptions are very important because they list the essential functions of your job, your duties and responsibilities, and your performance expectations. (Refer to the Appendix for a sample job description.) Be sure you know exactly what is expected of you. Watch for opportunities to excel and take advantage of them. If your company uses an evaluation form, ask for a copy. Make sure you understand the performance criteria and how performance is evaluated and scored. If your company uses computers to manage the different steps in the performance evaluation process, make sure you have the required computer skills. Keep a binder that includes "thank you's" from coworkers, patients, or physicians; awards or citations that you have received; transcripts of continuing education classes and courses you've completed; copies of professional certifications you've earned; and any other evidence of your performance and professional growth since your last evaluation. (This is valuable information to have at hand, not only for performance evaluations but also for applying for promotions. Keeping materials in a binder demonstrates your organizational skills.) Think about the goals you set for the past year. Did you accomplish them? Why or why not? Jot down your accomplishments and note what you would like to achieve in the coming year. Keep a list of questions you might want to ask your supervisor when you meet. If your company gives employees the opportunity to fill out a self-evaluation, take advantage of it. Evaluate your performance yourself and view it through the eyes of those with whom you have worked during the past year.

When the time approaches to meet with your supervisor, get a good night's sleep the night before and try to relax. (This is where being prepared really helps.) Expect some anxiety. Bring the file of documents you've collected all year long, your list of achievements and goals, and your self-evaluation. During the meeting, practice good listening skills. Take notes. Pay attention to everything your supervisor says and ask for clarification when necessary. In your own words, summarize what you think your supervisor is saying to avoid misunderstandings. If you disagree with something, state your reasons in an objective, respectful manner without becoming defensive. The purpose of these sessions is not to tell you what a bad employee you have been. The purpose of the evaluation and feedback session is to give you the information you need to become an even better employee. (Note: Please keep in mind that some supervisors are more experienced and skilled than others in providing constructive feedback and coaching their subordinates for improvement. Annual performance evaluations may create some uncomfortable conflict. Employees aren't the only people who experience anxiety over these sessions—many supervisors do, too.) Expect to hear some negative feedback. But if you've done your best all year long, you should also hear lots of positives! Accept constructive criticism and learn from it. Compare the score on your self-evaluation with the score determined by your supervisor and discuss any differences. If you have substantial disagreements with the content of your evaluation, most evaluation forms include a section for "employee comments." Be sure to state your opinions clearly and objectively. Don't expect the outcome of the evaluation to change, but at least you have had the opportunity to state your opinions. If you are expected to make improvements during the coming year, make sure you know exactly what's expected of you and how improvements will be measured. At the end of the session, summarize important "next steps" and thank your supervisor for the time he or she spent with you.

Remember—no one is perfect. We all have more to learn. Even if your company doesn't have a performance evaluation process, you can (and should) request periodic feedback. It can be as simple as asking, "How do you think I'm doing?" And you don't have to wait until annual review time to ask. Solicit feedback from your supervisor and coworkers on a regular basis and then act upon what they've told you. If your performance becomes an issue, chances are your supervisor will give you a "heads up" as soon as the problem becomes apparent. But don't subscribe to the "no news is good news" theory. Soliciting feedback from those most familiar with your performance is the best way to increase your value to the organization.

Compliance

Compliance with company policies and federal and state laws is extremely important. Ignoring a rule, violating a policy, or breaking the law can compromise quality, hurt a patient or coworker, or get you fired from your job.

What might happen if employees don't wear their identification badges at work? What if they ignore infection control precautions or leave confidential reports lying out in the open? What if they falsify documents or make threats against other employees?

Rules and policies are established for good reasons, and it will be your responsibility to follow them. Health care organizations usually have written policies and printed employee handbooks to communicate expectations. Know where to find these policies and, if you don't understand something, ask for clarification.

Corporate compliance is becoming an important topic in health care. Complying with federal and state laws and various internal and external policies and procedures has always been important. But compliance is gaining even more attention these days because the government is stepping up its efforts to identify violators and prosecute them. Hospitals and other health care organizations have begun creating new departments to oversee compliance issues. They're training employees to spot problems and report them. They're auditing individual departments to uncover and resolve any compliance concerns. Many companies are setting up hotlines so employees can make confidential phone calls to report compliance concerns anonymously with no fear of backlash.

Violating a law, regulation, or policy can get you and your employer in serious trouble. You could end up fired, prosecuted, fined, or incarcerated. Your employer could face stiff fines and exclusion from vital government programs like Medicare or Medicaid. Complying with laws, regulations, and policies because you have to is important, but there's more to it than that. Professionals comply because it's *the right thing to do.*

Make sure you're aware of, and understand, all of the laws, regulations, and policies that pertain to your job. Become familiar with medical/legal issues specific to your profession, the types of patients cared for, and the array of medical and other procedures you perform. Know where your organization stands on practicing sound business ethics and what is expected of you. If you're accused of an illegal activity, claiming "I wasn't aware of that law!" is not an acceptable legal defense. It's your job to know what laws, regulations, and policies apply to you and your work. If you're uncertain about any of them or unsure as to your own responsibilities, be sure to ask for clarification.

Some areas of risk that result in compliance concerns include patient confidentiality, safety and environmental precautions, labor laws, retention of records, Medicare billing and reimbursement, licensing and credentials, and **conflict of interest.** Examples of illegal or **unethical** behaviors include fraudulent billing (charging a patient for a test or treatment that he or she never received or intentionally coding medical procedures inaccurately), improperly changing or destroying records, personally profiting from self-referrals or insider information, **sexual harassment,** creating a **hostile workplace,** and stealing property.

Consider each of these issues and how it might affect your job. For example, always maintain the confidentiality of patient records, financial reports, and other materials that your employer deems private. Protecting patient confidentiality has become a major issue due to the widespread electronic transmission of medical information for insurance purposes. National standards referred to as **HIPAA** (the

Health Insurance Portability and Accountability Act of 1996) were enacted by the federal government to protect patients' personal health information from inappropriate use and disclosure. This set of rules ensures the patient's privacy. Keep in mind that you must have the patient's *written* consent for releasing information. Health care employers now include HIPAA training in their employee orientation sessions and students now receive HIPAA training in their educational programs. Make sure you know what is expected of you in order to comply with all HIPAA requirements. A failure to comply with HIPAA rules could result in fines up to and including $25,000. These fines can be imposed on the employer, individual employees, or both. No matter what your job may be, ensuring the privacy and security of medical information is paramount in health care. (Refer to the Appendix for additional information about HIPAA.)

Patients have legal rights that must be respected by all health care workers. In addition to personal privacy and confidentiality of medical records, patients also have the right to have family members or representatives of their choice and their own physician notified promptly of their admission to the hospital. Patients may formulate advance directives and expect to have health care staff comply with these directives. Patients may participate in the development and implementation of their plan of care, make informed decisions regarding their care, and refuse treatment. Patients have the right to receive care in a safe setting, free from all forms of abuse or harassment. Patient care must be free from seclusion and/or restraints of any form that are not medically necessary or are used as a means of coercion, discipline, convenience, or retaliation by staff. Patients may access their medical records within a reasonable time frame. In order to ensure these rights, health care providers must inform patients of their rights in advance of providing or discontinuing care, and establish a process for prompt resolution of patient grievances. It's very important to be aware of patient rights and your role in protecting and enforcing those rights.

There are far too many examples of compliance issues to list them all. Some of the most important include not modifying or destroying patient or financial records without proper authority. If your job involves billing the government or insurance companies for patient procedures, make sure the codes you use to identify specific diagnoses or procedures are accurate. Never up-code a procedure to increase reimbursement. Never accept pay for hours you did not work. Avoid any suggestion of a conflict of interest. For example, if your job involves awarding contracts to outside companies, don't accept gifts or free meals from a vendor in exchange for awarding it your company's business. Don't ask a vendor that your company does business with to give you a special discount on a personal purchase and don't refer patients to one of your relatives who just happens to be in the health care business!

Make sure you work within your **scope of practice.** Performing duties beyond what you're legally permitted to do is highly risky and illegal. Some jobs require a special **license** to practice. State agencies grant licenses only to people who have met pre-established qualifications, and only licensed workers may legally perform the job. Other jobs may require a special **certification.** State agencies and professional associations certify people who have met certain competency standards. Although noncertified people may legally perform the job, employers may prefer to hire only those workers who possess certification and who are eligible to use the professional title associated with that certification. When a license, certification, or some other special credential is required for your job, make sure you meet those requirements and maintain "active" status. In some professions this means completing annual continuing education requirements or periodic competency retesting.

Avoid any suggestion of unwelcome sexually oriented advances or comments that could lead to sexual harassment charges being filed against you. This includes verbal communication, visual and written materials, unwanted touching, or anything that has the potential to make another person uncomfortable. Even if you think your actions are harmless, the other person (or someone else present at the time) might see things differently. Never bring a weapon to work or create an environment where someone else could feel intimidated or unsafe. Verbal threats, nasty letters, inappropriate cell phone photos or voice mail or text messages, or other forms of hostile behavior may lead to charges of intimidation.

As a professional, you would never knowingly engage in an illegal or unethical act yourself, but you might observe someone else doing something suspicious. Or you might feel that you are a victim of sexual harassment or a hostile work environment yourself. If you have a concern about something you see going on at work that might put you, your employer, your coworkers, or your patients at risk, be sure to let your supervisor know or report your concern via a hotline if one is available. If your supervisor is one of the people involved in the activity, report the matter to your supervisor's boss, to a human resources representative, or to someone in legal services. If you feel you're the victim of sexual harassment or intimidation, report the incident to your supervisor or another superior immediately. It's wise to keep written documentation of what you've observed or experienced, including details such as the date, time, place, who else was present, and a description of what exactly happened and what you did to follow up. Information like this will be very important during an investigation.

If you know someone else is engaged in illegal behavior, it's your responsibility to report it. If you don't, you could get in trouble, too. In fact, even if you didn't know but should have known, you can be liable for legal action. For example, if you observe someone stealing from patients, report it immediately. If you don't report it and your supervisor finds out that you knew what was going on, you could be disciplined. If your job involves maintaining an inventory of supplies and a coworker gets fired for stealing some of them, you could get in trouble for not noticing that items were missing. Keep on your toes and stay alert! If you find yourself in a situation where you aren't sure how to proceed, ask yourself some questions. Is what's going on legal and ethical? Is it in the best interests of my employer and patients? How would this look to others outside my organization? Then take action.

You've probably heard the term **whistle blower**—a person who notifies authorities when another person or a company is involved in wrongdoing. Blowing the whistle can be a scary proposition for employees, but the law protects whistle blowers from retribution. In fact, whistle blowers might receive a portion of the fines the government collects from health care organizations found guilty of Medicare fraud, for example. If you suspect someone of illegal or unethical behavior, it's your responsibility to report it. It's best to try to get your concern resolved within your organization first. Avoid going to the government or to the media unless repeated attempts have failed. If you've tried your best to report and stop illegal or unethical practices but have been unsuccessful, you might need to think about finding another job.

Representing Your Employer

When you accept a job offer, show up for work, and receive a paycheck, you become a representative of the company. To patients, visitors, guests, and vendors, you are that company. Everything you do and say can have an impact on the company's reputation. By accepting employment, you not only agree to follow your company's rules and policies but also agree to support its mission and abide by its values. What is your employer's **corporate mission?** What are the company's **corporate values?** What should you do to support the mission and values?

Learn everything you can about your company so you can talk intelligently about it with others in the general public. Read company newsletters and keep up on the latest events. Even though you don't own the business, it's still your company, so take an interest in it. You're an important part of the company you work for and you have an obligation to get involved and support your employer. This begins with the language you use. When referring to your employer, avoid words like *they* and *them*. Instead, use *we* and *us*. For example, instead of saying "They told us they will open the new clinic next week," it's better to say, "We're opening our new clinic next week." It's not *they* did something or *they* said that, it's *us* and *we*. Take some pride and "ownership" in the company you work for. It's part of being a professional.

Regardless of what job you will have, your appearance, attitudes, and behaviors reflect the company you work for. **Front-line workers** such as nurses, medical assistants, radiographers, housekeepers, phlebotomists, patient transporters, and food service workers have some of the greatest influence on the company's reputation because they have the most frequent contact with patients, visitors, and guests. What might happen if you openly criticize your employer or complain about a company policy in public, or if you question how a physician, nurse, or other caregiver treated a patient? By damaging the reputation of your employer, you're hurting yourself and countless other employees who come to work each day to do a good job. If you have complaints or concerns, there are appropriate ways to communicate them inside the organization. Don't make negative remarks about your company or its employees in public. Use **discretion** and be careful what you say and to whom you say it. Give your employer and your coworkers the benefit of the doubt and assume that everyone is there to do his or her best. If you have serious doubts about your employer and the way your company does business, it's probably best to find another job.

Understanding the importance of professionalism, knowing where you fit into the big picture in health care, demonstrating a strong work ethic, improving quality, complying with laws and policies, and representing the company you work for in a positive manner are all important aspects of being recognized as a professional. The next step is examining who you are *as a person* to see how your personal values and character traits support professionalism in the workplace.

L E A R N I N G   A C T I V I T I E S

Using information from Chapter One:

❏ Respond to the What If? Scenarios below

❏ Answer the Review Questions below

❏ Watch the video for Chapter One on the accompanying Student CD-ROM and complete the CD-ROM Assignments

What If? Scenarios

Think about what you would do in the following situations and record your answers.

1. You were out with friends until very late last night and had to report for work this morning at 7:00 a.m. You know your coworkers won't arrive for another half an hour. You've got just enough time for a quick run to the corner coffee shop before your coworkers arrive.

2. You promised your coworkers you'd work the day shift on Thanksgiving so they could be home with their families. Then two days before the holiday, an old friend from out of town calls to say he'd like you to be his guest for lunch on Thanksgiving Day.

3. You have an appointment with your supervisor next week to review the results of your annual performance evaluation. You overhear one of your teammates telling another person that she gave you a low score on your 360-degree feedback evaluation because you refused to trade shifts with her over Thanksgiving weekend.

4. Your shift ends in 30 minutes and you've got about 30 minutes of work left to do, but you haven't gotten to take your afternoon break yet.

5. Your supervisor asks you and two of your coworkers to proofread a financial report to make sure the calculations are accurate. Your coworkers have already reviewed the document and found no errors. You waited until the last minute to start reviewing the material and now it's time for you to go home.

6. You overhear a purchasing agent talking on the telephone with a salesperson from a local computer company. She offers to buy 15 new computers for your company if the salesperson will also agree to sell her son a computer at the same quantity discount.

7. The office manager tells you to enter a code on an insurance claim form that she knows is not correct. If you enter the incorrect code that she tells you to, the clinic will receive more money from the insurance company than it would if you enter the correct code.

8. One of your neighbors is admitted to the unit where you work. A relative of yours calls to tell you he's heard a rumor that the neighbor has a communicable disease. Because you work on the unit and have access to records, your relative asks you to find out if the rumor is true.

9. A new piece of equipment gets installed in your department, but you miss the in-service session when everyone gets trained on how to operate it. The next day there's a procedure to be done using this equipment and it's your responsibility to do it.

10. A coworker invites you to a party. When you arrive, you notice three other people that you work with complaining about low wages and telling a group of strangers that one of the surgeons at your hospital made a mistake in surgery last week and lied to the patient's family to try to cover it up.

Review Questions

Using information from Chapter One, answer each of the following.

1. Identify three factors that positively impact recognition as a health care professional.

2. List eight health care jobs that are important and require professionalism.

3. Explain the importance of a systems perspective.

4. Identify five factors that demonstrate a strong work ethic.

5. Differentiate between the terms *accountable, reliable,* and *diligent.*

6. Describe the attitudinal differences between optimists and pessimists.

7. Define *corporate compliance, conflict of interest*, and *whistle blower.*

8. Discuss the importance of confidentiality and HIPAA.

9. Identify how competence and scope of practice impact quality of care.

10. Define *corrective action* and list five behaviors that could result in job dismissal.

11. Explain the purpose of performance evaluations and list three ways to prepare for one.

12. Differentiate between objective and subjective evaluation criteria.

CD-ROM Assignments

Select Chapter One on the Student CD-ROM and complete the assignments.

chapter two

Personal Traits of the Health Care Professional

"The person that loses their conscience has nothing left worth keeping."

Izaak Walton, Writer, 1593–1683

"The ultimate measure of a man is not where he stands in moments of comfort and convenience, but where he stands at times of challenge and controversy."

Martin Luther King, Jr., Civil Rights Leader, 1929–1968

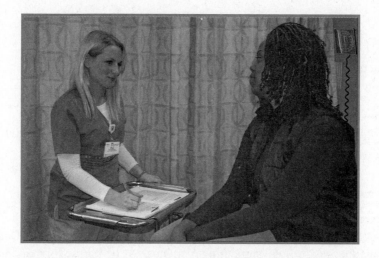

Professionalism in Action

The Student CD-ROM that accompanies this book contains video scenarios and other learning activities related to this chapter. Once you complete reading this chapter, turn to the CD-ROM to gain a richer understanding of the concepts presented here.

Chapter Objectives

Having completed this chapter, you will be able to:

- Define *character* and *personal values* and explain how these affect your reputation as a professional.
- List four examples of lack of character in the workplace.
- List four examples of positive values in the workplace.
- Explain how character, personal values, and priorities define who you are as a person and how you conduct your life.
- List three important questions to ask yourself when making difficult ethical decisions.
- Discuss the importance of your word being as "good as gold."
- Give three examples of dishonest behaviors and describe the impact of dishonesty in the workplace.
- Define *ethics* and *morals* and discuss how they impact decision making and behavior.
- Define *fraud* and give three examples.
- Define *reputation* and list three factors that influence a person's reputation.

Key Terms

character

conscience

ethics

fraud

integrity

judgment

morals

personal values

priorities

respect

reputation

trustworthiness

Character and Who You are as a Person

As mentioned in the Introduction, professionalism brings together who you are as a person and how you contribute those traits in the workplace. Before you can achieve success "doing" something, you have to "be" something and being a health care professional depends greatly on who you are as a person. It takes a long time to develop a good reputation and only a split second to lose it. Much of this comes down to your core **character** and your **personal values.**

Webster's New World Dictionary of the American Language, College Edition, defines *character, values,* and *reputation.* Character is an "individual's pattern of behavior or personality," a "description of the traits or qualities of a person," the person's reputation, and his or her "moral constitution." Personal values are those things that have a "high degree of worth" to the individual, that are "highly desirable and worthy of esteem." A person's character and values give direction to one's behavior and ultimately result in one's **reputation**—"character in the view of the public or community, whether favorable or not."

Employers are becoming increasingly concerned about a lack of character and positive personal values in the workplace. Each year in businesses throughout the country, employees are responsible for stealing millions of dollars worth of goods from their employers and from other employees. Hidden video cameras in hospitals reveal employees stealing computers, office supplies, syringes, medications, and patients' personal possessions. Employees captured on videotape are sometimes caught sleeping on the job, watching television, or engaging in sexual activity with a coworker. Would-be employees falsify information on job applications and over-state their education and work records. Countless numbers of fraudulent workers' compensation claims are filed each year. Arguments, fistfights, workplace violence, and sexual harassment are becoming more commonplace. Billing personnel rou-tinely up-code claim forms to increase insurance reimbursement. Managers are increasingly involved in conflict-of-interest situations.

It's no wonder that employers are placing more and more emphasis on the char-acter of their employees to help reduce theft, absenteeism, dishonesty, workplace vio-lence, substance abuse, safety infractions, negligence, and low productivity. Increasingly, employers are hiring for character, praising for character, and pro-moting for character. Character reflects a person's **morals**—the capability of dif-ferentiating between right and wrong—and it influences **integrity** and **trustworthiness,** two key factors in professionalism.

How do character, values, reputation, morals, integrity, and trustworthiness apply to you as a person? How do they affect the way you approach your work? Do you know the difference between right and wrong? Are you honest? Can you be trusted? If you make a bad decision, can you overcome it and get back on track?

Reputation

No single factor is more important in being recognized as a professional than a per-son's reputation. As mentioned earlier, it takes a long time to develop a good repu-tation and only a split second to lose it. After years of being an honest, law-abiding individual, all it takes is one dishonest act or a single incident of unprofessional behavior to shake people's confidence in you and lose their trust. This is why pro-fessionals must work hard each and every day to do what's right and to maintain the trust and respect of others.

If you've developed a pattern of behavior over the years based on lying, cheat-ing, stealing, and taking advantage of other people, then changing your character at this point in your life is going to be quite a challenge, but the potential is there. Our sense of acceptable behavior starts at a very young age when our parents and other influential people in our lives begin to teach us the difference between right and wrong. As children, we experiment with different kinds of behavior to see what reactions we get. If those who raised us believed in discipline, we soon learned the consequences of "doing something bad." We were taught to get along with other children, to share our toys, to wash our hands before we eat, and to clean our rooms and make our beds. Unacceptable behavior resulted in "getting grounded" and losing privileges like playing outside with our friends or watching a favorite television program. Over the years, we learned to make **judgment** calls, to compare our options and decide which is best. We learned the concept of self-control and the importance of avoiding temptation. Through relationships with other people, we learned about fairness, respect, **ethics,** and loyalty. We learned to care, to give, and to appreciate. And before long, our character, values, and **priorities** began to define who we are as people and how we conduct our lives.

Judgment and Decision Making

As adults, we're faced with multiple decisions every day—what to do, why to do it, how to do it, when to do it, where to do it, with whom to do it, and so on. Some of the decisions we must make are "small" ones—what to eat for breakfast, where to go for lunch, who to invite for dinner. But other decisions, especially those involving relationships with people, require much thought and carry significant consequences—how to resolve a disagreement, when to say "no," whom to ask for help.

Many questions must be considered when making decisions: What are my choices? How do the options compare with one another? What might happen? Who might be affected? How would it make me feel? How would my decision be viewed by other people? When the decisions you face involve your job, more questions arise: What would my supervisor think? How would my coworkers feel? Could I lose my job?

Most people have a **conscience**—a little voice that gnaws away at you, keeps you from sleeping at night, and constantly says, "You *know* this *isn't* the right thing to do!" Your conscience can be quite reliable in reminding you of the differences between right and wrong. When you're facing some really difficult ethical decisions, even more questions need to be considered. How would this look if it appeared in the newspapers? How would my children feel? Would my family support me? Could I look myself in the mirror? Would I be able to sleep at night?

The problem is that some people either have no conscience, have learned to ignore their conscience, or have become good at rationalizing their behavior. It starts with something small, like telling a lie or stealing some candy, and then grows and grows until it becomes a way of life. Eventually, dishonest and unethical behavior will be revealed but, in the meantime, countless people may be victimized.

The good news is that the majority of Americans are honest, law-abiding people with good character and sound moral values who sincerely want to do what's right in their lives. They face temptations but summon up the courage to say "No!" and they don't engage in dishonest behavior just because "everyone else does." People become angry with someone else but later revert back to compassion and forgiveness. They look out for themselves but still treat other people with fairness and respect. At times everyone needs some help exercising good judgment. But for the most part, the majority of us make the right decisions for the right reasons.

In the health care workplace, personal traits like character, values, morals, ethics, integrity, and trustworthiness are absolutely vital! If you were sick or injured, what kind of people would you want caring for you? If you owned a health care business, what kind of people would you want working for you? Let's take a closer look at character traits that are most essential for recognition as a health care professional.

Respect and Trust

A big part of professionalism is earning people's **respect,** which starts with their ability to trust you and the quality of the decisions you make. In today's society, we've become increasingly suspicious of other people. "Don't trust anyone!" is common advice. Unfortunately, that perspective gets reinforced each time we set ourselves up to believe in someone or depend on someone, only to end up disappointed or let down. The previous chapter discussed the importance of reliability and following through when someone is counting on you. When your word is as "good as gold," your supervisor and coworkers know they can trust you to (1) be there when you're supposed to be, (2) perform the responsibilities of your job with competence, and (3) keep your promises and meet your obligations. Once trust is established and maintained over time, respect will likely follow. If you promised to give a coworker a ride to work, don't forget to pick him or her up. If you received training on a new procedure and your supervisor is trusting you to perform it properly, make sure you know what you're doing. If you tell a patient you'll relay a message to her nurse, follow through. If you want people to respect you, make sure you can be trusted.

Honesty

Earning respect also relies greatly on being viewed as an honest person. As mentioned earlier, dishonesty has become highly visible in the health care workplace. The cost of health care is high enough without employers having to pay for extra supplies, food, and equipment stolen by its employees. Most health care workers would probably deny that they steal from their employers or patients. But theft goes well beyond stealing a computer or a patient's wallet. For example, if you manipulate your time card and get paid for more hours than you actually worked, that's theft. If you sleep on the job, take unauthorized breaks, or leave your work area without permission and still receive pay for that time, that's theft. If you make personal long-distance phone calls on a company phone, that's theft. If you use garage passes for yourself that were meant for visitors and guests, that's theft. If you take a sandwich off of a dietary catering cart waiting to be delivered to a luncheon meeting, that's theft. If you take supplies off of a patient's bedside table for yourself to use at home, that's theft. Anytime you take *anything* that doesn't belong to you without proper authorization, it can be construed as theft. Is a "free" sandwich or box of cotton swabs worth losing your job over? What about an extra hour of pay that you didn't really deserve? This is where both honesty and good judgment enter the picture. Even if taking something that doesn't belong to you appears totally harmless, what might be the consequences?

The same is true with lying and cheating. Both are dishonest behaviors that can get you in big trouble. Little, seemingly harmless, "white lies" usually snowball into big, complicated lies that can become difficult to manage. Lies are eventually uncovered and, before long, people will wonder if they can believe *anything* you say. Being truthful is always the best approach and sometimes telling the truth takes courage. For example, what if you witness two coworkers leaving work early one afternoon after writing in a later time on their attendance sheets. If your supervisor notices their absence and asks if you know their whereabouts, what would you say? Would you be tempted to lie and say "No, I don't know where they are?" After all, you have to work with these two people every day, and if you "squeal" on them, they might make life hard on you later on. As just mentioned, telling the truth takes courage and you're going to have to make decisions like this one on a regular basis. So let's examine the matter more closely. First of all, let's look at your coworkers. If you lie for them, will *they* respect *you?* Does it matter? After all, your coworkers are dishonest. They're falsifying records and stealing from the company—*your* company. Is their opinion of you so important that you're willing to lie for them? What about your supervisor? You could probably tell this lie and get away with it, but what if he or she found out? Is protecting the secrecy of dishonest coworkers worth losing your job? Then there's you and your conscience. Who can you be sure will know you've told a lie? You, of course! If you tell this little "white lie" and get away with it, what's next? When you see someone stealing a syringe from the supply room, are you going to lie for that person, too? After all, syringes aren't all *that* expensive and there are plenty left. Would you lie for someone stealing a computer? How about stealing personal possessions from a patient? Just where are you going to draw the line?

Listen to your conscience. You know what your coworkers did was wrong. And you know if you lie to your supervisor, that's wrong, too. So summon up the courage and tell the truth—and get a good night's sleep! If you do make a bad judgment call and tell a lie, have the courage to admit it and accept the consequences. Corrective action or getting dismissed from your job would be a big price to pay for your dishonesty, but at least you'd learn a valuable lesson.

Cheating is an example of dishonest behavior that can result from giving in to temptation. Maybe you have a test to take and didn't have time to study. It would be so easy to just stick some notes in your pocket and refer to them during the test. After all, you can go back over the material later—after you've passed the test. If your instructor or supervisor finds out that you've cheated on the test, you'll be in big trouble. You could fail the course, lose your job, or both. And if you think your classmates will stand by quietly and let you get away with cheating, think again. They put in the time to study for the test and you didn't. As with stealing, cheating goes well beyond what you might typically think of. For example, if you use information from someone else's report and then call it your own work, that's cheating. If you're given too much change in the cafeteria line and you keep the extra money, that's cheating. If you call in sick when you really just want a day off, that's cheating. Can you cheat just a little and get away with it? Ask your conscience.

A very serious example of dishonest behavior is falsifying information, also known as **fraud.** As mentioned in the previous chapter, fraud is not only dishonest, it's illegal. Misrepresenting your education, credentials, or work experience on a job application, résumé, or other document is fraud. Billing an insurance company for a patient procedure that never occurred is fraud. Backdating a legal document, entering incorrect data on equipment maintenance records, or changing the results of a research study are all examples of fraud. As with stealing and cheating, there may be more to fraud than you realize. If you sign someone else's name without his or her permission, that's fraud. If you turn in a time card that's inaccurate, that's fraud. If you tell your supervisor you passed a competency assessment when you really didn't, that's fraud. Being convicted of fraud not only can cost you your job, it can cost you your freedom, too.

Ethics and Morals

Two other character traits that factor into recognition as a professional are your ethics and morals. Both play a major role in decision making and behavior. Do your ethics and morals support professionalism? For example, would you let someone outside your company borrow your ID badge so he or she could get an employee discount on purchases in the gift shop? Would you satisfy your curiosity by sneaking a peek at a confidential file that contains your supervisor's annual salary? Would you skip work on a day when you knew your unit would be exceptionally busy? Would you threaten to report a coworker's mistake unless he or she covers your shift for you on the next holiday? Would you date a coworker and then share the intimate details at work? Would you place an anonymous phone call to a local television station to get a coworker in trouble? Would you clock out for your best friend so she could leave early? Would you ask a coworker to clock out or lie for you?

If it seems like some of the examples of ethical and moral issues overlap with those involving lying, cheating, stealing, and other dishonest acts discussed earlier, your observations are correct. When it comes to dishonesty, it's hard to separate one type of unprofessional behavior from another. For example, failing to return the extra change to the cashier in the cafeteria line is not only cheating, it's theft. Sneaking a peek at your supervisor's salary is not only unethical, it's a breach of confidentiality. Clocking out for a friend is not only unethical, it's fraud.

The point is that every decision you make and every action you take can have a huge impact. One bad judgment call can erode someone's trust in you. One unethical decision can destroy your reputation. One illegal act can cause you to be fired from your job—or worse.

If you find yourself in a difficult situation weighing one option against another, and you're not quite sure which course of action to pursue, consider the following questions: Is it honest? Is it ethical? Does it reflect good character? Is it based on sound moral values? How would it affect my reputation? Would it damage the trust others have in me? Would I be respected for my decision? What would a professional do? What does my conscience tell me to do? What impact would my actions have on others?

This chapter could continue on with more examples of how character and values reflect on who you are as a person and how your personal traits affect decision making and behavior in the workplace. But you already know what kind of person you are and you know the difference between right and wrong. You also know what's expected of health care professionals. Either you can choose to live up to those high standards, or you can try to slide by with less. No one can make that decision for you. If you make some poor decisions now and then and stray from the behavior expected of professionals, it's important to make some changes in your life and get back on track.

Chapter Three explores personality types, communication skills, and teamwork as preparation for working with coworkers, patients and their family members, and other types of customers.

L E A R N I N G   A C T I V I T I E S

Using information from Chapter Two:

❏ Respond to the What If? Scenarios below
❏ Answer the Review Questions below
❏ Watch the video for Chapter Two on the accompanying Student CD-ROM and complete the CD-ROM Assignments

What If? Scenarios

Think about what you would do in the following situations and record your answers.

1. You witness a coworker taking money from the petty cash box in your department. She says she needs to borrow the money to get her car fixed and she'll pay it back when she gets her next paycheck. She reminds you that she did you a big favor when you first started your job and asks that you not report her to the supervisor.

2. You need to have your time card signed by the end of the day. You know your supervisor would sign it, but she's tied up in a meeting and your shift ends in 10 minutes.

3. You have one more paper to turn in for a course you're taking that's required for your job. You keep the weekend open to write it, but an old friend calls and says he'll be in town for the weekend and would like to spend it with you. You know there won't be enough time both to write the paper and to visit with your friend. You just happen to have a copy of a paper that someone else wrote for the same course two years ago that earned a grade of "B." The course is being taught by a new instructor who would never know that you didn't write the paper yourself.

4. Your supervisor asked you to attend a meeting in her place but you forgot to go. You know she'll be upset with you because she needs the information that was handed out. Someone else you know did go to the meeting and has agreed to give you copies of the handouts. When you hand the information to your supervisor, she asks, "So what did you think of the meeting?"

5. A patient on your unit gets discharged. While cleaning the room for the next patient, you find an expensive watch in the drawer in the bedside table. It's a woman's watch and the former patient was a man.

6. When you open up your paycheck, you realize that you got paid for a day that you didn't work.

7. You'd like to call your sister in Maine but can't afford the long-distance phone charge. The phone in your break room has long-distance access and other workers have used it for personal calls without being questioned.

8. As a research assistant, your salary and the project you're involved in are funded by a federal grant. If the results of the research are positive, the grant and your job will get renewed for another year. The director of the research project asks you to help him change some of the data to indicate better results.

9. When it's time for your annual competency evaluation, your supervisor announces that you and your coworkers will be checking each other off. Your coworkers get together and decide just to give each other a satisfactory evaluation without actually checking each person's competency level.

10. Your son and daughter are returning to school tomorrow after summer break. You haven't had time to shop for school supplies and are short on cash right now. Your company is overstocked with office supplies and no one would miss a few pencils, pens, and tablets of paper.

Review Questions

Using information from Chapter Two, answer each of the following.

1. Define *character* and *personal values* and explain how these affect your reputation as a professional.

2. List four examples of lack of character in the workplace.

3. List four examples of positive values in the workplace.

4. Explain how character, personal values, and priorities define who you are as a person and how you conduct your life.

5. List three important questions to ask yourself when making difficult ethical decisions.

6. Discuss the importance of your word being as "good as gold."

7. Give three examples of dishonest behaviors and describe the impact of dishonesty in the workplace.

8. Define *ethics* and *morals* and discuss how they impact decision making and behavior.

9. Define *fraud* and give three examples.

10. Define *reputation* and list three factors that influence a person's reputation.

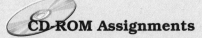

CD-ROM Assignments

Select Chapter Two on the accompanying Student CD-ROM and complete the assignments.

chapter three

Working with Others

"The dictionary is the only place that success comes before work. Hard work is the price we must pay for success. I think you can accomplish anything if you're willing to pay the price."

Vince Lombardi, Football Coach, 1913–1970

"We make a living by what we get, but we make a life by what we give."

Winston Churchill, British Prime Minister, 1874–1965

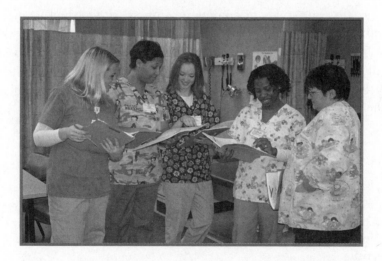

Professionalism in Action

The Student CD-ROM that accompanies this book contains video scenarios and other learning activities related to this chapter. Once you complete reading this chapter, turn to the CD-ROM to gain a richer understanding of the concepts presented here.

Chapter Objectives

Having completed this chapter, you will be able to:

- Describe the concept of interdependence and list three techniques to strengthen teamwork and interpersonal relationships.
- Explain why coworkers should be treated as customers.
- Discuss two ways to demonstrate loyalty to your coworkers and your employer.
- Identify four types of workplace teams and explain how they differ.
- Discuss how personality differences can cause conflicts in the workplace.
- Define *diversity,* list five examples of cultural differences, and explain why it's important to have a diverse health care workforce.
- Explain the role of respect, good manners, and courtesy in the workplace.
- Describe why communication skills are the basis for effective relationships.
- List three problems that may occur when communicating electronically and describe three ways to prevent them from happening.
- Define *conflict resolution* and explain its importance.
- List the four styles of communication, identify which is most effective in conflict resolution, and describe the potential impact of each style.
- List four types of customers found in health care settings and give five examples of good customer service.
- Describe five ways to provide good customer service for hospitalized patients and their family members.

Key Terms

body language	intradisciplinary teams
cliques	intradepartmental teams
colleagues	interdepartmental teams
conflict resolution	interdisciplinary teams
consensus	loyal
diversity	manners
empathetic	multiskilled
group norms	self-esteem
heterogeneous	self-worth
homogeneous	synergy
inclusive	work teams
interdependence	project teams
interpersonal relationships	

Interpersonal Relationships with Coworkers

Now that we've examined character traits and how they're applied in the workplace, it's time to discuss how health care professionals work with other people. How you interact with other people and the relationships you form with coworkers are the basis for success in the workplace. **Interdependence** is a key element in providing direct patient care and the many support services that comprise our health care system. No one person can do it all. Only groups of people working together can get the job done and done well.

Professionals devote a lot of energy to establishing positive **interpersonal relationships** and they treat one another in a caring, respectful manner. How you work with your colleagues helps mold your reputation as a professional. Valuing diversity, good manners and social skills, and effective customer service and interpersonal communication skills are all key factors in a professional work environment. Let's look at each of these to see how you get along with other people.

If you're employed on a full-time basis, you probably spend as much time with your coworkers each day as you do with your family and friends. Nothing can make your job more pleasant or miserable than relationships at work. Think about the relationships you've had with people in the past. What made those relationships work or not work? People want to feel good about coming to work and getting along well with others helps create a positive, enjoyable work environment.

Effective relationships are based on many of the factors discussed in the previous chapter—trust, honesty, ethics, and fairness. But working well with others requires several additional traits and interpersonal skills. For example, health care professionals are well-versed in customer service techniques. Did you know that your coworkers are your customers, too? That might sound odd, but your coworkers are your "internal" customers. They deserve to be treated with the same respect and compassion that you would give your patients. Apply the same communication skills, conflict resolution techniques, and manners with your coworkers that you would use with other customers.

An important part of effective interpersonal relationships at work is creating and maintaining a positive attitude and always looking for the best in situations. Professionals have an optimistic outlook. They "see the glass as half full, not half empty." They see opportunities and challenges, not just problems. They look for the best in people, give others the benefit of the doubt, and assume everyone is there to do his or her best. It's important to be viewed as a team player, to cooperate with others, and to contribute to the team effort. Smile every chance you get; say "hello" when you meet people in the hallways; and avoid creating a negative environment by whining, complaining, and questioning authority. Complainers "poison" the workplace and stir up discontent. If you get labeled as a complainer, you'll be viewed by management as a troublemaker and your opportunities for advancement will be limited or nonexistent.

Be **inclusive.** Rather than excluding people and participating in **cliques,** invite people to join you and welcome their friendship. How do you feel when you're left out of a group? Excluding people can hurt their feelings. Keep in mind that you have a great deal of influence on how other people feel about themselves. A person's **self-esteem** and **self-worth** result, at least in part, from the feedback he or she gets from others. Help people recognize their strengths and abilities, support their growth and development, and celebrate their accomplishments with them.

Because health care workers are interdependent, it's important to share information openly. Unfortunately, some people hoard information because it gives them a sense of power over others. They have something you don't and it makes them feel important. An attitude like this is counterproductive to teamwork. Also share space, equipment, and supplies. Remember, you and your coworkers are all there for the same purpose—to serve your patients and other customers. There's no need for competition. Laugh at yourself, be a good sport, and maintain your sense of humor. Avoid arrogance and don't be a snob. Never "look down" on other people or treat someone in a demeaning way because he or she has less education, income, or "status" than you. There will always be people "above" you and "below" you in the hierarchy of your organization, and *every single person* is important in accomplishing the company's mission. Remember the "golden rule" and treat others as you want to be treated yourself. Gain satisfaction from your accomplishments and feel proud, but don't brag. Always acknowledge the achievements of others and credit their efforts.

Building effective relationships doesn't happen overnight. It's hard work and you have to hang in there. Be patient with yourself and with others and be forgiving. No one is perfect—not even you! Get to know people better—you may see a whole different side of someone's personality and the many priorities he or she must balance. Let your coworkers get to know you better, too. When you know your coworkers well and form strong relationships, you may be in a better position to anticipate one another's needs and be willing to help.

Part of professionalism and earning the respect of others is being **loyal** to those who have helped you. Health care professionals work in stressful environments. Part of interdependence means coworkers must be able to rely on one another for encouragement and emotional support. This is extremely important when the going gets rough. Sometimes it can be difficult to get the kind of emotional support you need from those who don't work in health care themselves. Even though family and friends want to help you, unless you've been there yourself, it's hard to relate to the stress of working with sick and injured people every day—and especially with critically ill children and patients who are near death. Professionals are there for one another, to lend a helping hand or a shoulder to cry on. When someone you work with needs support, be ready to help. Most times it means just listening—and understanding.

The discussion about loyalty also relates to the relationship between you and your employer. Chapter One mentions that "*you* are the company you work for."

When you think about it, you don't actually work for a company, you work for the *people* who manage the company. After all, companies are just legal entities that own assets such as buildings, property, and equipment. You don't work for a building, you work for people! Professionals make that distinction and they feel a sense of loyalty to the people they work *for* as well as those they work *with*. Even if you don't agree with all of management's policies or you feel as if you deserve more pay or better benefits, remember that management is providing you with employment and an opportunity to make a living. What can you do to demonstrate your appreciation for and loyalty to your employer? Of course, the most important thing is to always give your job your best effort and provide excellent customer service. Whenever you get the chance, express your appreciation to management and let managers know it makes you feel proud to be a part of the company. Managers and administrators are people, too, and they appreciate being appreciated. If your employer invests in your education and helps you acquire some new skills, pay the company back. How can you do that? By continuing to work for the company for a reasonable length of time after training rather than taking your new skills across town to go to work for the competition. A local competitor might offer you some extra pay to "jump ship," but remember who invested in your education to begin with and demonstrate your loyalty. Someday you might need a letter of recommendation from your current employer. If management views you as a loyal employee, it can only help.

Loyalty is based on relationships that benefit all parties involved. Establishing strong interpersonal relationships with your coworkers creates a more positive, supportive environment in which to work. Offer to help someone else even if he or she has not asked you for help. When you've got a tough job to do or you're running late, isn't it a welcome relief to have someone walk up to you and say "Need a hand?" Be willing to rotate shifts and holidays—your coworkers will appreciate such consideration. Be willing to make personal sacrifices for others while keeping your own needs in mind. Sensitivity and kindness are rewarded many times over.

Learning to rely on one another is vital, especially in emergencies and other stressful situations. Gain an appreciation for the strengths, abilities, and personal traits that make each individual unique. Be familiar with contributions that others bring to the workplace so everyone can count on one another when the need arises. Volunteer to serve on committees to meet people from other areas and to establish relationships with them, too. Sign up for employer-sponsored classes and recreational activities. Join people during your lunch break and widen your circle of **colleagues.** You'll find there's **synergy** in working with other people. A group can accomplish so much more than people working independently as individuals.

Relationships with colleagues can enrich your life, but your coworkers do not necessarily need to be your friends. Friendship is not the goal of respectful collegial relationships. You might not even like some of the people with whom you work, but you should respect their knowledge, skills, and the talents they bring to the workplace.

Teamwork

One of the most important aspects of interpersonal relationships is teamwork. Team-work helps to build and promote pride in your work. Health care organizations are becoming increasingly dependent on teams and teamwork. In fact, many hospitals and other types of health care facilities rely on "high-performance work teams."

Depending on your profession and where you work, you will likely participate on many teams during your health career. **Intradisciplinary teams** are composed of employees in the same discipline, such as radiographers, medical assistants, or surgical technologists. Team members have similar educational backgrounds, job duties, and scopes of practice. Because of the similarities among team members, intradisciplinary teams are also referred to as **homogeneous.** Sometimes team members all work in the same department and other times they work in different departments. A team of radiographers, for example, might include staff from main radiology, the emergency department, and outpatient services, all working together to resolve issues or make improvements. **Interdisciplinary teams,** on the other hand, are composed of employees from different disciplines. Team members have different educational backgrounds, job duties, and scopes of practice. Due to team member differences, interdisciplinary teams are also referred to as **heterogeneous.** Interdisciplinary team members may work in the same department or in different departments. A team of medical technologists, phlebotomists, and nurses might meet together to better coordinate specimen collection, labeling, and processing among staff on patient care units and the clinical laboratory. **Intradepartmental teams** are composed of employees from the same department or work unit. Sur-gical nurses, surgical technologists, and instrument technicians, for example, might form a team to improve instrument sterilization and packaging. **Interdepartmental teams,** on the other hand, are composed of employees from two or more different departments. Representatives from the information technology, admitting, and patient registration departments might meet to streamline patient registration processes. Two other types of teams are **work teams** and **project teams.** Work teams meet on an on-going basis as part of their jobs. A group of paramedics, for example, might meet weekly to monitor patient transport and quality outcome data. Project teams, however, meet for a specified period of time and disband when their project has been completed. Some projects are short-termed (such as creating a new electronic form for patient documentation) while others occur over a longer period of time (such as creating a new computerized database to track patient discharges.)

As a health care professional, it's not necessary to "label" the teams you're on, using the terms in this text. What is important is your ability to serve as an effec-tive team member. Team members benefit from extra training in interpersonal and communication skills, negotiation and conflict resolution, delegation, and valuing diversity. "High performance work teams" work independently with little direct supervision. Management creates the team, identifies the members, arranges for meeting times, communicates expectations, and clarifies the team's assignment. The team itself then takes over at that point. Self-directed teams may be charged with arranging their own work schedules, determining holiday coverage, selecting new equipment and medical supplies, monitoring and improving quality outcomes, and resolving budgetary and staffing issues. When a vacancy occurs, teams may interview and select new team members. With 360-degree feedback performance evaluations, team members help evaluate the performance of their teammates. As you might imagine, effective communication and interpersonal skills are absolutely vital when serving on teams with responsibilities such as these.

Whether you are a part of intra- or interdisciplinary teams, intra- or interdepartmental teams, work- or project teams, or homogeneous or heterogeneous teams, you must become skilled at both "leading" and "following." You will probably find yourself in both roles, even within the same team. "Shared leadership" is becoming more common. This means that members of the team all share the responsibility of "leading" as appropriate. Each team member leads the others when the task to be completed falls within his/her unique area of expertise or interest. For example, you may serve on a team to develop a dress code for your department. The assignment includes: reviewing dress codes from other departments, facilitating group discussions to get staff input, meeting individually with vice presidents to get executive input, drafting the new dress code policy, and then "defending" the policy at a department-wide staff meeting. Which of these steps in the process would you want to lead? The team might divide up responsibilities based on each team member's expertise, personal preferences, experience, and availability. Some people are "born leaders" and effective communicators. They emit confidence and are comfortable leading group discussions, even when the conversation includes disagreements and controversy. Other people prefer the "follower" role, panicking at the thought of having to speak in front of a large group of potentially angry coworkers. But the team member who's comfortable in the follower role during this phase of the assignment might "take the lead" in drafting the new policy and sitting down with executives to get their opinions. In shared leadership, there's usually a role for each team member to play, taking advantage of each person's strengths and experience. The key is to know yourself and your team members well and to divide up and share leadership responsibilities according to individual attributes and the willingness to serve. The information on personality preferences presented later in this chapter will help.

Providing leadership on a team is not the same as "supervising" team members. In many cases, team members are considered peers with one another. No team member "reports" to another team member. But if one member of a team fails to complete his/her responsibilities adequately, the whole team may suffer. Perhaps you have already experienced situations such as this while working on group projects as a student. In some companies, team performance is just as important as individual performance. When the team performs well, each member is held in high regard. When the team fails, each member is held accountable. As a team member, participate actively. Complete your assignments on time. Perform your share of the workload and follow through. Share communication openly. Cooperate and provide assistance. Don't just identify problems—help solve them. Serve as both leader and follower. Your success depends on the success of your team.

Employees who work in teams are often cross-trained to function as **multiskilled** workers. This means they're capable of performing more than one function, often in more than one discipline. For example, a housekeeper might be cross-trained to perform basic maintenance and repair duties. A nursing assistant might learn to draw blood and prepare specimens for laboratory analysis. A unit secretary might learn to admit patients and process bills. A maintenance worker might also acquire carpentry skills. Multiskilled workers who participate on teams tend to be highly productive. They can provide more services than individuals working independently and can enhance convenience for patients. They bring versatility and flexibility to the staffing plan and they save the company some money in labor costs. Cross-training has become a major trend among health care employers and it's likely you will encounter this concept in your work, too.

Whether you work with the same team on an ongoing and daily basis, or with a variety of different teams to tackle short-term projects, team skills are vital for health care professionals. Think about some of the teams of which you've been a member. Which teams worked well together and which ones did not, and why? Serving on a team can present all kinds of challenges and it requires some special skills. Having to achieve **consensus** when agreement is called for can be a big challenge. Consensus is more than just "voting" on different options and "majority rules." With majority rules, there are winners and there are losers—the majority wins and the minority loses. The objective of consensus, however, is to arrive at a win-win resolution. Through group interaction, team members strive to select an option that *all* members agree to support. As you might imagine, that can be quite a challenge. But setting up win-win situations and operating by consensus are the underpinnings of good teamwork. Good communication skills are absolutely essential—a topic discussed later in this chapter.

Developing effective teamwork takes time, especially among diverse groups of people with different personalities, values, and communication styles. But being part of a smooth-running team can be one of the most exhilarating experiences for health care professionals. Work with your teammates to establish **group norms**—guidelines that can help the group function well. This includes such things as: (1) Every member is expected to participate in decision making, (2) each person's opinion will be listened to and respected, (3) all members will do their share of the work, and (4) no one may leave for the day until the team's work has been completed.

If you acquire the skills needed for effective leadership and "followership" and incorporate the behaviors you are learning in this text, you will thrive on teams and reap the benefits of collaborating with others to achieve remarkable results.

Personality Preferences

Just as you are a unique individual with your own personality and preferences, so are all of the other people with whom you come in contact. Personality types vary widely and they influence how people interact with one another and how they participate (or don't participate) in a group setting. Personality types also influence how people size up situations, make decisions, and approach their work.

Learn as much as you can about your own personality type and gain some insight into the personality types of the people with whom you work. The more you know about someone's personality, the better you will understand that person and be able to work with, and communicate with, him or her. There are many personality assessments available. One of the oldest and best known is the Myers-Briggs Type Indicator (MBTI). The MBTI provides an accurate, reliable method for identifying and comparing differences in personality preferences. A valuable feature of the MBTI is the research that's been conducted to demonstrate how different personality types can best work together in the workplace. The MBTI can help you learn more about your own personality type and those of the people with whom you work. Some people are "what if?" types. They like to brainstorm, use their imaginations, and come up with new ideas. What if? people have difficulty actually implementing a new idea because, once the idea has been conceived, they would prefer to move on to thinking up the next new idea rather than continuing to work on the original one. On the other hand, people with the opposite personality type don't enjoy the What if? phase. They prefer having someone else come up with the idea and then turn it over to them to coordinate the implementation phase. Obviously, you need both types of people to come up with good ideas and get them implemented. Another way the MBTI looks at personality differences is via the introvert/extrovert. Introverts prefer to work alone in a quiet setting without distractions. Extroverts prefer to work in an open group setting with frequent interactions with the people around them. Some people base their decisions on logic and analysis. Others base their decisions on emotions and feelings. If you're interested in learning more about personality types, check with your advisor or counselor for information on how to access assessments like the MBTI. Keep in mind that there is no "right" or "wrong" when it comes to personality types—just differences. Learn all you can to help identify these differences and then use them to everyone's advantage in the workplace.

Diversity

Differences among people extend well beyond personality types and preferences. Other examples of **diversity** include differences in gender, age, race, culture, ethnic background, lifestyle preferences, religious beliefs, socioeconomic status, and physical condition. The United States is a multicultural nation, composed of people from different cultures with a variety of personal values, communication styles, and work ethics. Professionals learn how to work with all kinds of people and to make the most of differences. Learning to work with people who are different from you presents some challenges but can also be quite rewarding. Diversity presents opportunities to take advantage of our differences and use them to everyone's benefit.

The workplace requires a variety of people to get the work done. For example, if you're helping to write a new policy for your department, you might look at the situation differently than someone who is much younger or older than yourself. A young, single woman might have a different perspective than an older, married man. Someone from a Latino culture might place a greater value on a particular issue in the policy than someone from an Asian culture. All points of view must be taken into consideration to accommodate our diverse population.

In health care, another type of culture is the occupation in which you work. Registered nurses, for example, have a culture based on their educational background, where they work, what functions they perform, and the knowledge and abilities they possess. Physicians have a culture too, as well as pharmacists, medical technologists, secretaries, surgical technologists, maintenance workers, and environmental services personnel. In health care organizations, there's a hierarchy based on these cultures and sometimes it causes problems. As mentioned earlier, cross-training has become a major trend in health care. Because multiskilled workers are trained to provide more than one function, they often work in more than one area. They may encounter multiple cultures and may not feel totally accepted or comfortable in any of them. This is also true of workers referred to as "extenders." Examples are patient care assistants (PCAs) or patient care technicians (PCTs). PCAs and PCTs are not nurses but they work alongside nurses in assistive roles. Because PCAs and PCTs have less education than registered nurses (RNs), function at a lower skill level, and lack RN credentials, they aren't a part of the RN culture. Often called "unlicensed assistive personnel," PCAs and PCTs may experience some difficulty fitting in and feeling like a part of the team. The same may be true for housekeepers, transportation aides, phlebotomists, and other types of non-RN workers assigned to work on patient care units. This also occurs in other areas, too—anytime someone "different" enters the group. Extenders can be found at other levels of the health care hierarchy, too. Physician assistants, for example, are physician extenders. Health care teams are composed of workers from different occupational cultures. Surgical teams, for example, include surgical technologists, surgical nurses, surgeons, and anesthesiologists. Surgical teams are supported by the efforts of schedulers, surgical attendants, instrument technicians, and others. Each type of worker has a different education level and scope of responsibility but all of them play important roles in the operating room.

Experiencing a hard time fitting in and being accepted by other cultures are common problems in dealing with diversity. But do differences *have* to pose such difficult challenges? Think about it. Does it really matter if your coworkers are younger or older than you, of a different gender, or from a different race or ethnic group? Does it really matter if some have more or less education than you or are skilled in a different health occupation? All of you have to work a little harder to get to know each other better and to figure out the best way to not only accommodate your differences but to make them work to the group's advantage. The point is, you're all there for the same purpose—to provide high-quality health care. Focusing on the mission of patient care gives diverse groups of workers some "common ground" to build on.

If you find yourself in a situation where you've been placed in a culture that feels uncomfortable to you, hang in there. Learn as much about the other cultures as possible and let others learn about yours. Let people know what you're capable of doing. Establish trust, build strong relationships, and work hard to develop a team spirit. Remember the earlier discussion about inclusion. When someone from a different culture is placed within your culture, do your best to make him or her feel welcome. Avoid passing judgments on other people. Whether we like to admit it or not, human beings have prejudices. Consciously or subconsciously we form opinions based on what we've seen, heard, read, or experienced. Prejudices begin in childhood and develop as we're growing up. Our environment, educational experiences, families, and friends all influence our beliefs and how we view people who are "different from us." As adults and as health care professionals we must be open to new ways of thinking and seeing the world through other people's eyes.

The world would be a simplistic, boring place if we were all alike. Diversity is an absolute necessity to the health and wellbeing of our planet and those who inhabit it. As health care professionals, we serve the complete array of a diverse patient population. In an ideal world, the health care workforce would reflect that diversity as well. By now you've read a great deal about the need for interdependence. Everyone working in health care needs everyone else to get the job done and done well. And our patients need all of us.

Respect

Diversity and respect go hand in hand. Regardless of whether you're working with people just like yourself or different from yourself, respect is the basis for getting along well with others. Once you understand how people differ from one another and you realize that there are no "good" people or "bad" people—just different people—you can learn to respect everyone regardless of his or her differences.

Think about yourself. If your personality, culture, or opinions are different from those of another person, don't you still want that person to respect you? People have a right to be different and to exercise those differences because we live in a democracy. You have a right to your opinions and other people have a right to theirs, assuming that laws are not violated and no one gets hurt or victimized in the process. Your job as a professional is to respect differences and the people who possess them. Show respect for everyone regardless of job title, background, cultural heritage, and so forth. Go out of your way to be especially kind to people who work in service and support roles. The "health care culture" places great value on its highly educated, professionally credentialed clinical caregivers such as RNs and doctors. Service and support workers often feel they're at the bottom of the ladder. All too often, they're treated as if they're almost invisible. As a result, they sometimes feel underappreciated and taken for granted. Acknowledge their efforts and let them know how much you value the work they do. Until you've walked in someone else's shoes, you have no idea all that his or her job involves. The same is true for people who are "above" you on the occupational ladder. You may see highly educated, professionally credentialed people failing to give subordinates (including you!) the credit they deserve. Try to give them the benefit of the doubt and don't take their lack of appreciation of your efforts personally. Health care personnel, especially physicians, function under a great deal of stress. But stress is not an excuse for inappropriate behavior. A curt remark aimed at you might not have anything directly to do with your own performance. If you do your best and show respect and appreciation for the efforts of others, your professionalism will speak for itself.

Draw on your character traits to show your respect for others. Be sincere and sensitive to other people's needs. Be considerate, kind, and sympathetic. Never ridicule someone, embarrass, or make them "feel dumb." Don't participate in gossip, pry into people's personal affairs, or be judgmental about how someone chooses to live his or her life. Respect the choices that other people make, even when you don't understand those choices yourself. If someone tells you something in confidence, maintain that confidentiality.

Respect a person's determination to do something on his or her own without your assistance. When people come to you for advice, be honest and remember how much influence you might have on the decisions they make. Respect people's privacy, personal possessions, and space. Respect people's health—don't come to work sick and spread your germs to others. Respect people's time and don't keep them waiting unnecessarily.

Keep your personal matters personal and avoid dealing with personal problems while you're at work. If you must make a personal telephone call, keep your voice low so you don't distract other people around you. Better yet, wait for a break and use a telephone outside your work area. Don't allow your personal pager or cell phone to interrupt others at work. Don't chatter away mindlessly about non-work-related topics and interrupt other people from getting their work done. Don't bring things to work to sell and don't spend work time buying things from other employees. Always respect the fact that people come to work to get things done. It's good to practice your social skills with coworkers—but only during breaks and after hours.

If you're having a problem with a particular person and an attitude, behavior, or action he or she has taken, show respect by discussing the situation directly with the person first. Avoid taking matters to a supervisor until you've tried to resolve the problem yourself. If someone were having a problem with something you did, wouldn't you appreciate him or her coming directly to you first rather than to your boss?

Always respect authority. Even if you dislike your supervisor as a person, or you find fault with his or her job performance, it's still important to show respect for his or her experience and position within the organization.

Manners

Often, demonstrating respect comes down to having good **manners.** As young children, most of us learned manners from our parents and from other influential people in our lives. But all too often in today's society, manners and common courtesy fall by the wayside.

Manners are standards of behavior based on thoughtfulness and consideration of others. Be aware of, and sensitive to, other people's needs. Courtesy and small considerations can make a big difference. For example, ask others before adjusting the temperature of the room or playing music on the radio. Return borrowed items as soon as possible and in the same condition as when you borrowed them. If you break something you've borrowed, repair it or replace it at your own expense. Don't expect other people to clean up after you. Keep your own work area neat and orderly so it doesn't become an eyesore for others. Avoid putting up risqué calendars, posters, or other personal items that might offend someone else.

Say "please," and always acknowledge your appreciation when someone does something nice for you by saying "thank you." When someone has done something really special for you, send him or her a thank you note or small gift. Use your company's employee recognition program to recognize the "beyond the call of duty" efforts of your coworkers. When someone you know joins a group you're with, introduce that person to the others. Be kind to strangers and try to make them feel welcome. Listen while other people are talking and don't interrupt them.

Hold doors open for people. When you see someone struggling to carry something heavy, help them. If you notice someone who looks lost, ask if you can help him or her find the way. Practice good elevator etiquette. If several people are waiting for an elevator, let the others go first and wait for the next one. If you're riding on an elevator with a patient on a cart or in a wheelchair, protect their privacy and don't stare at them. If you're in a crowded room with limited seating, offer your seat to someone else. If your supervisor or a coworker invites you to lunch as his or her guest, don't order the most expensive item on the menu. When going through a banquet line, make sure you leave enough food for those in line behind you. If you're invited to a meeting or another event that involves a meal, be sure to notify the person organizing the event as to whether or not you'll be attending.

Good manners and common courtesy are just "common sense" for health care professionals. Watch for opportunities to display good manners with everyone you encounter and set a good example for others.

Communication Skills and Conflict Resolution

Just because you have good interpersonal skills, treat people with respect, and use good manners doesn't guarantee you'll get along with every person in every situation. In fact, you can pretty much count on some interpersonal conflicts with the people you work with. First of all, everyone's working in a stressful environment. When you're under pressure or feeling rushed, you don't always practice your best communication skills. And second, because of the diverse types of people you encounter, you cannot help but experience some difficulties getting along with everyone. You don't have to be best buddies with each and every coworker. In fact, there may be a few people you'd rather not work with at all. But because you can't choose your coworkers, and you can't change them either, you must find a way to get along with one another. Good communication skills can really help. How effective are your communication skills? Are you good at **conflict resolution** and confrontation?

Communication is extremely important in teamwork and interpersonal relationships. You must be able to communicate effectively to get along with people and to complete your work appropriately. Communication is a two-way process. Messages are sent and received. Both aspects of the process must work well to support good communication. But, unfortunately, much of what is communicated is misunderstood. When communication breaks down, it's often because the person receiving the message isn't listening well to the person sending the message. Good listening skills are vital. It's important not only to *listen* to someone but also actually to *hear* what that person has to say. Most of us need to improve our listening skills. Learn to listen carefully and concentrate on the message so that you fully understand the other person's point of view. Repeat what he or she has said in your own words to make sure you received the message accurately. It's tempting to only "half-listen" while you're thinking about how you are going to respond. But if you do that, it's likely you'll miss part of the message. Always ask the other person for clarification when you don't fully understand what he or she is saying. Or ask the person to state the message again in different words. Observe the person's **body language**—the nonverbal messages—to gather more information. A great deal of information is communicated nonverbally. This includes eye contact, "rolling" of the eyes, posture, hand gestures and body movement, tone and loudness of the voice, facial expressions, and so forth. Body language often communicates more information, and a greater accuracy of information, than the actual words you use.

Hone your skills at sending messages to other people. Be clear and concise and use terms your listener can easily understand. Think about the vocabulary you use and make sure your terms are not unfamiliar or of too high a level to be understood. Give examples as further explanation. Don't get frustrated if the other person just "doesn't seem to get it." Hang in there and keep trying. If the conversation seems to be going nowhere, ask a third person to help out.

In today's highly technologic world, communicating electronically by email, voicemail, cell phone, text mail, computer, telephone, and fax offers efficiencies and convenience. But electronic communication also creates the need for caution, especially when using email and voicemail. With email, the receiver sees only the words that you have written. Without actually hearing or seeing you, the message becomes somewhat impersonal. The "tone" of your message (i.e., serious, humorous, sympathetic) could easily be misunderstood or misinterpreted by the receiver. You may have sent a humorous message, but the receiver might have interpreted your communication as serious. As mentioned previously, body language often conveys more information than the words used. Had you delivered your message in person, your body language would have communicated "humor," not "serious." When delivering messages by voicemail, the receiver hears your words *and* your tone of voice, but your body language is still invisible. When you need to be absolutely certain that your message has been conveyed and received accurately, it's best to speak with the person face to face. The second best option is a live telephone conversation.

Another disadvantage of communicating by email is accidentally sending a message to the wrong person or people. If you are a frequent user of email, you've probably already made this mistake and hopefully learned a lesson. Either you mistakenly clicked on the wrong address, sent the wrong message to the wrong person, or forwarded a previous message to another person without realizing what you were doing. Similar problems may occur with voicemail messages. Anyone who receives a voicemail message from you may forward that message to someone else. These types of situations can be highly embarrassing and may accidentally reveal sensitive, confidential information to people who should not have access to it. When communicating electronically, slow down and think about what you are doing. Make your messages short and to the point. Omit information that could become problematic if it falls into the wrong hands. Exercise care when forwarding previous messages. Before you click on "send," double-check the content of the *entire* message and confirm to whom it is being sent.

With email communication, you cannot always be certain the message was received and read. Electronic communication isn't foolproof. At work, people receive scores of email messages every day. Sometimes messages are deleted accidentally without being read. People become overwhelmed and never open all of their messages. Some people with access to email never use it. Keep in mind that electronic communication leaves a documented "trail" of messages. If you're angry with someone and send an emotionally charged message by email or voicemail, the receiver has documented evidence of your communication and could use it against you. If you had had a live telephone conversation with the person or met with him/her in person, there would be no documented communication record. With both email and voicemail, even if you have deleted a message, it's still retrievable electronically. Deleting electronic messages does not mean they are gone forever. Always stop and think before you send any electronic message. Do you really want to send a message when you are angry or emotionally upset? How would you feel if a message ended up in the wrong hands?

Computer security is a major issue in today's world. Protect the security of your passwords, don't share passwords with anyone, and avoid using the same passwords at work that you use at home. Many companies require employees to change their passwords on a regular basis. Security can be compromised, so the potential exists that non-authorized people could gain access to your email correspondence and your company's private and confidential information. Be sure to follow company policies that protect the security of computer systems and confidential information. Failure to do so could result in a breach of confidentiality, a violation of HIPAA laws, and embarrassment for you and your employer. Also, avoid checking your personal email messages at work and don't spend time surfing Internet sites that are not related to your work. Employers usually have policies stating that company computers are for business use only. Accessing inappropriate web sites at work can result in your termination.

You've no doubt heard the phrase "dealing with difficult people." Responding to confrontation, confronting people yourself, and resolving interpersonal conflict all require some special communication skills. There are four basic styles of communication: aggressive, passive, passive-aggressive, and assertive. Let's examine an example of each style and see which one works best in confrontation and resolving conflicts. You and a coworker both want Christmas Day off. Both of you have relatives arriving in town and wish to spend time with them. After discussing the holiday schedule, it becomes obvious that one of you must work.

Using an *aggressive* style of communication, tone of voice, and the body language that goes along with it you say, "I've worked here longer than you so I deserve this day off! Besides, you don't have any children and I do!" Your coworker replies, "You got Thanksgiving Day off and I had to work. So I deserve Christmas Day off more than you! And besides, your children are adults now and my grandchildren are coming in for Christmas!" You reply, "Why do you always have to insist on getting your own way? Every time we do a schedule, you complain!" "I complain?" your coworker responds. "You're the one who always refuses to work overtime!" You can imagine where the "conversation" goes from here. With aggressive communication, the conflict usually gets worse. The sender (you, in this example) expresses his opinion honestly but does so in a way that fails to show respect or consideration for the receiver. The receiver (your coworker, in this example) becomes defensive and fights back. Before long, anger has taken over, other issues enter the conversation, and the conflict escalates into aggressive behavior. Situations involving aggressive communication can turn violent and shouting or fistfights might occur. The conversation can be overheard by others, including supervisors and patients. Did anyone "win" in this situation? Was the conflict resolved? It's clear the answer is "no." Let's try a different approach.

Using a *passive* style of communication, you say, "Well, I guess if you want Christmas Day off, I'll go ahead and work. Maybe my kids can come back for Easter and I can spend some time with them then." With passive communication, the sender (you) fails to express his or her opinion openly and honestly and displays little self-respect. You just turn into a floor mat to be walked on! The receiver "won." He got his needs met. But the sender "lost." In fact, you come off looking and feeling pitiful. Was the conflict resolved? In a way "yes," but over the long run you will likely feel resentful of the other person and disappointed in yourself for not standing up for something that was important to you. Let's try again.

Using *passive-aggressive* communication, you say, "Well, I guess if you want Christmas Day off, I'll just have to work. Maybe my kids can come back for Easter and I can spend some time with them then." Then, as soon as you get the chance, you do something sneaky to "get even." Maybe you send your supervisor an anonymous note saying your coworker takes longer breaks than he's supposed to. You spread malicious gossip about the coworker behind his back. Or you call in sick on a day when the two of you are assigned to work together. After all, there are lots of ways to get even. Maybe doing so will make you feel better, maybe not. With passive-aggressive communication, the sender (you) still fails to express his or her opinion openly and honestly and displays little self-respect. But then, to make matters worse, you do something sneaky or dishonest. Was the conflict resolved? No, not really. Let's try one more time.

Using *assertive* communication, you say, "Well, we both want the day off. I'm sure you'd like to spend Christmas Day with your grandchildren. After all, you had to work Thanksgiving, didn't you? On the other hand, because I've worked here twice as long as you, I do have seniority. And my children are really looking forward to spending the day together as a family. So let's figure out a way to work this out so we can both get our needs met." Maybe you could split the holiday shift. Maybe you could arrange a long weekend off to make up for one of you having to work the holiday itself. Maybe you could work together to find a third person willing to cover for both of you. There is almost always a reasonable solution to every problem. But if you're arguing with another person, your energy is spent on the conflict, not the resolution.

With assertive communication, the sender (you) states his or her opinion openly and honestly but in a way that shows respect and consideration for the other person. This presents the best opportunity for both people to work together, to compromise, and to come up with a solution that's acceptable to both of you. It's a win-win situation—which is the goal of conflict resolution. It's also good experience for honing your problem-solving skills.

After reading this book up to this point, it should be obvious that assertive communication is the only acceptable communication style for health care professionals. You must have enough self-respect to state your needs openly and honestly. You must not allow yourself to be "walked on," pitied, or tempted to do something underhanded and sneaky to get even. Professionals look out for themselves but do it in a way that shows respect for the needs and desires of their coworkers.

Assertive communication doesn't come easy—it takes practice. Maybe you're not used to standing up for yourself when someone confronts you or disagrees with you. Maybe aggressive or passive-aggressive communication has been your style up until now. If so, it's time to start working on a different communication style that's more appropriate in the workplace. Put some effort into developing your assertive communication skills. Observe how other people deal with conflicts and the results they get. Then keep practicing your own skills. The more you practice, the easier it will become.

Learn to "choose your battles wisely." Decide which conflicts are really worth tackling and which ones you should just "let go." Some battles aren't worth the effort. And be careful! Just because you're taking an assertive approach, there's no guarantee the other person will, too. Someone may turn aggressive on you. When confronting a "difficult" person, make sure you can get out of the room quickly if you need to. If there's any concern about your physical safety, make sure there is someone else nearby who can come to your aid if necessary. Remember, it's a crazy world out there. You never know when someone might be carrying a weapon or behaving in an aggressive or passive-aggressive manner.

When you decide to confront someone, make sure you have all the facts first—complete and accurate information. Give the other person the benefit of the doubt until you've fully investigated the matter. Don't proceed on assumptions that may not be true. Don't rely on unverified, third-hand information. Don't go off "half-cocked" only to regret later something you've said or done. Stay calm, keep your anger and tone of voice in check, and arrange a suitable time and place to discuss differences. Never conduct this type of conversation in a public area. You may be able to control your own behavior but you cannot control the behavior of the other person. Listen carefully and make sure the other person understands your point of view, too. Aim for a win-win situation whenever possible. Once you fully understand the other person's point of view and he or she understands yours, there should be a middle ground where both of you can compromise and feel like your needs have been met.

When you have a conflict with a coworker, resolve it quickly. Procrastination only makes things worse. But calm down first and make some rational decisions about how to handle the matter. Attack the issue, not the person. Remember that you cannot change other people; only they can change themselves. All you can do is make your best effort at communicating appropriately. If necessary, ask another person with good conflict resolution skills to serve as an intermediary.

If one of your superiors is the "difficult person," proceed cautiously! Remember to respect his or her position of authority. Weigh the pros and cons of addressing the situation head-on or just learning to live with it. If you decide to discuss the matter with your superior, plan in advance what you're going to say, how you're going to say it, and what response you'll give to how he or she might react. Practice delivering the message in advance and consider role-playing the situation first with someone you trust. Listen carefully, watch for a win-win resolution, and be open to receiving some constructive feedback that might help you form a more positive relationship with your superior in the future. If the matter is still unresolved and you cannot adjust to accepting it and moving forward, consider talking with a human resource representative or another person in authority in your department. If the situation is serious and cannot be resolved, you may need to transfer into another position.

Effective communication and conflict resolution skills will serve you well in all aspects of your life. Avoid letting other people "press your buttons." When you hear yourself saying, "She makes me so angry!" stop and think about that statement. You have a choice as to whether to be angry or not. Allowing other people to "make you" angry means you are giving power over your own behavior to the other person. Is that really what you want to do? Find ways to maintain control of your own behavior and don't allow other people to push you into doing things or saying things that you would rather not do.

Before moving on, a few more comments need to be made about communication skills. So far, we've focused on verbal communication because of its importance in interpersonal relationships. But no discussion of communication skills would be complete without also addressing nonverbal communication, written communication, public speaking skills, and grammar.

As mentioned previously, nonverbal communication is the message you send by way of body language, eye contact, facial expressions, gestures, and so forth. You can convey your anger, disappointment, or frustration with someone without even saying a word. Similarly, you can allow yourself to be taken advantage of by slumping in your chair, cowering in the corner, or avoiding eye contact with the person with whom you are communicating. As with assertive communication, watch how other people use good or poor nonverbal communication skills. Observe their strengths, weaknesses, and the results they get. Think about your own nonverbal communication and how it can be improved.

The ability to communicate well in writing is certainly important and most everyone can benefit from sharpening his or her writing skills. Even if your job doesn't involve extensive writing, how you express yourself through written communication still has an impact on being recognized as a professional. Poor written communication skills can impede advancement in your career. If you struggle with writing, spelling, or punctuation, get some help. Take a course, do some self-study, or work one-on-one with a basic skills instructor. Make sure you can record accurate telephone messages, write clear notes to coworkers and your supervisor, and construct basic memos and letters should the need arise. If your job involves recording data on charts or other kinds of forms, make sure your writing is legible and your entries are accurate. If writing reports or preparing handouts for meetings is part of your responsibility, you'll need some higher level writing skills to help you organize information and present it in an appropriate format.

Spelling is important, especially in health care. With medical terms, changing just one letter in a word can change the entire meaning. If you fill out forms to order tests or treatments for patients, order patient supplies, or process bills or other kinds of paperwork, make sure you can spell terms correctly.

Few challenges in life are more anxiety-producing than having to get up in front of a group of people and make a presentation. But public speaking skills are important, especially if your job requires you to give updates at meetings, make announcements to the rest of the staff, or teach coworkers something new. Becoming comfortable with public speaking is like facing any other fear—the more you do it, the better you'll get, and the more comfortable it will become. Start out small, with a group of supportive people, and build from there. And remember, most of the people in the audience will be glad it's you up there instead of them!

Grammar is also an important aspect of good communication skills. This topic will be addressed in the next chapter dealing with your image as a health care professional.

Customer Service

The remainder of this chapter discusses interactions with coworkers, physicians, vendors, guests, patients, and visitors—all of whom are considered customers of the health care industry. Depending on your job, you may deal with some or all of these different types of customers. The factors that define effective interpersonal relationships with coworkers also apply to customer service and how you relate to the people with whom you come in contact each day. Some people cringe at the thought of referring to patients as "customers" or "consumers." But keep in mind that health care companies are businesses, too. It's important that customers are pleased and satisfied with the services they receive. A growing number of health care companies use the term "service excellence" instead of "customer service" and they devote significant time to "service excellence" or "standards of service" training for employees.

Like coworkers, your customers are a highly diverse group of people. They represent all personality types and a wide variety of differences. Some will be easy to get along with and others will be more difficult. Some will be downright nasty. Some will appreciate your efforts whereas others will not. But all customers deserve to be treated with respect and good manners.

Effective communication skills and conflict resolution techniques are extremely important in customer service. Equally important is knowing what it takes to "satisfy" customers and maintain that satisfaction. Let's start with a closer look at patients as customers.

The grades you earn in school are important. But it doesn't matter if you were a straight A student if you can't, won't, or don't behave like a professional when interacting with patients. Possessing sufficient knowledge is important, but applying what you've learned in your interactions with patients is where "the rubber meets the road." Everyone, patients included, expects you to be competent. That's just "a given." What sets you apart as a professional is how you behave. Working in direct patient care is a privilege. It's an honor to have another person entrust their health and safety to you. It's also an awesome responsibility. Today's patients have high expectations regarding how they will be treated by health care workers and they have choices as to where to obtain health care services. Patients won't hesitate to go someplace else for their care if they believe they haven't been treated well.

When you work in direct patient care, the patient should be the focus of everything you do. It's not about you, your department, or your schedule for the day. It's *always* about the patient. When you arrive for work, remember this. Today is just another typical day for you. But for your patients, it could be a day that they will never forget. Assuming they live to see another day, they will tell scores of people about their experience and how they were treated. Patients don't miss much—they hear and notice everything going on around them. If there's tension among the staff, they pick up on it. If a piece of equipment doesn't work, the rest room hasn't been cleaned, or the lettuce on the cafeteria salad bar is rotting, they notice. Patients spend a lot of time (too much time) waiting. It's amazing how much information a patient can acquire just sitting in a waiting room or lying on a cart headed for surgery. If you think the patient can't overhear your phone conversation halfway down the hall, think again.

When people become patients, they're vulnerable and at their worst. Some are literally scared to death. They're in pain and anxious, worried, confused, and overwhelmed with the medical experience. Many patients feel helpless, having to turn themselves over to people who will make decisions about their care. They're concerned about what might happen to them, how their lives will be affected, how their children and spouse will fare in their absence, and a whole host of other issues. Patients need reassurance and confidence that they are in good hands. How you look, communicate, and behave can have a tremendous impact on their feeling of security.

Every thing you say and do has an affect on patients. Small acts of kindness on your part may be huge to patients. Patients and family members pick their favorite caregivers. Upon returning, they may ask to have the same person who took care of them the last time take care of them again. Some caregivers "go the extra mile" and those are the ones we want our patients to remember. These professionals "connect" with and "engage" with people. They're able to filter out everything else going on around them and concentrate on "being there" at that precise moment for that patient. The connections that professionals make with their patients are not the result of "acting" or "performing a duty." They're a reflection of the caregiver's personal values and professional priorities, an indication that caring for others comes straight from the heart. Isn't this the kind of person you want providing health care for yourself and your loved ones?

Remember what you've learned about valuing differences and diversity. These concepts apply to patients and other customers, too. It's not your place to be judgmental. Regardless of whether a patient is wealthy, poor, homeless, elderly, a transvestite, or a criminal, each one should be treated with respect. Respect their privacy and the confidentiality of their personal and medical information. Protect their dignity, self-respect, and personal possessions. Refer to patients as "Mr." or "Ms." Avoid terms of endearment such as "honey," "sweetie," and "dear." Be compassionate, caring, and **empathetic.** Anticipate your patients' needs and be prepared to meet them. No request or concern is too trivial. However, if a patient asks you for a drink, food, medication, or assistance walking to the rest room, never fulfill the request yourself unless your job includes these duties. Always refer any matter that is outside of your scope of practice to the patient's nurse or another caregiver on the unit and then make sure the appropriate person follows through.

When communicating with patients, use terms they can understand. If they ask you a question you are not capable of answering or are not authorized to answer, refer the question to the appropriate person. Never read a patient's medical record unless it's part of your job. Never divulge information about a patient's medical status to the patient's family members, clergy, or other visitors without the patient's permission. Confine the exchange of confidential information to a "need to know" basis when discussing patients with other health care professionals. If you have patients who are celebrities, leaders in your organization, or coworkers, make sure you protect their privacy and give them every consideration you would give other patients. Never ask questions or make comments in a public area that might embarrass a patient or violate privacy. For example, a medical assistant should never raise his or her voice to ask Mr. Jones, who is sitting in the public waiting area, whether he remembered to bring his stool sample! Avoid the temptation to give your own personal opinion when a patient asks, "Which doctor in this group is the best?" or "Which doctor would you take your child to?" Don't discuss your own medical history or conditions, or that of your family members, with patients. Always stop and think—if *you* were the patient, how would you want to be treated?

No discussion of customer service would be complete without mentioning the patient's family members and close friends. A patient's family is his or her "lifeline" to their normal life. When the patient invites other people to be a part of his or her medical experience, these other people become part of the patient's "team." Patients need families and friends to help them through difficult situations. Having clergy present may help. Sadly, not all patients have a support system. Some patients will complete their entire hospital stay with no family present or any visitors. These patients need some special compassion and attention from their caregivers. Other patients have large families and lots of friends. Policies regarding hospital visiting hours have always been controversial. Some hospitals strictly enforce limited visitation while others have abandoned visitation limitations altogether. The problem is that visitors don't always use common sense. If a person is sufficiently sick or injured to require hospitalization, then he or she needs rest and shouldn't become tired with too many visitors. On the other hand, maintaining connections with family and friends is an important part of the healing process. Sometimes it's up to the caregiver to enforce some visitation limitations to carry out the wishes of the patient and what's best for his/her recovery.

Families of seriously ill patients may literally "camp out" at the hospital. They want to be as close to their loved one as possible, and for as much time as possible. Spouses may spend the night in their loved one's room, even though it's very uncomfortable. Families bring things from home to comfort them and the patient, such as favorite foods, flowers, and personal items. They may bring clothes and toiletries because they are "living there" for the time being. The patient's room could become cluttered with people and things. Try to avoid viewing this as an inconvenience to you and remember—this is the patient's and his/her family's "home away from home" for the time being. Providing family support is an important part of customer service and patient care.

As mentioned earlier patients notice everything. When a patient is hospitalized for several days, the patient and his/her family spend hours and hours, and days and days, waiting. Their lives are on hold until their medical situation is resolved and they can resume their normal routine. With so much time on their hands, they notice when the free coffee down the hall isn't strong enough, the upholstery on the chairs is threadbare, and the elevator doors close too quickly. When it's finally time to eat, there's never an extra wheelchair available to push grandma down to the cafeteria. The patient's room is too hot or too cold. The meal tray was supposed to be delivered 20 minutes ago and when it finally arrived, the milk was white instead of chocolate. The TV remote control doesn't work right. Patients and families become irritated when they don't get medical information about the patient's condition and treatment plans quickly enough. Doctors make rounds on the patient care units when it's most convenient for them. Families will stay in the room all day and refuse to leave even for meals for fear of "missing the doctor" when he/she makes rounds. They'll pressure you for information that you don't have and ask for answers that you cannot give. It's enough to make a sane health care worker crazy! Please try to give your patients and their family members the benefit of the doubt and remember that their lives are in limbo. They're temporarily living in suspended animation, in some surreal world, usually not by choice. They're uncertain about what's going to happen next and no one has all of the answers. Take a deep breath and remember why you went into health care. Give them some slack and rejoice that *you*, unlike your patients, get to go home in a few hours.

Avoid the temptation to give personal advice or to express your own religious beliefs. When appropriate generate some humor and laughter. Be positive whenever you can. Even tiny improvements in the patient's condition mean a great deal to the patient and his or her family members. Here's where your optimistic "the glass is half full" attitude can be helpful. Perhaps the patient's blood pressure and heart rate haven't settled down during the past hour. But they haven't worsened either. Maybe the patient isn't well enough to be transported to radiology for a chest x-ray. But he can sit up in bed and have a portable radiograph taken in his room. Maybe the patient's IV supply can't be completely disconnected, but the dosage has been reduced. Look for things to be happy about and express them. Optimism and a positive outlook on the part of caregivers are important to patients. A positive frame of mind can lead to improvements in a patient's condition. When undergoing high-risk procedures, patients who are optimistic and more relaxed may have better outcomes. If a patient thinks his or her medical team has given up, he or she may give up, too. But don't give patients "false hope" or get their "hopes up" inappropriately. Some of your patients won't get better. Some won't leave the hospital alive. As stated earlier, working in direct patient care is a privilege. You may have the opportunity to help prepare someone for death. The patient and his or her family will have difficult decisions to make. They will need privacy and time to talk, cry, and express their love and other emotions. They may have to "say goodbye" as the cart is wheeled out of the room on its way to surgery, facing the prospect of never seeing their loved one alive again. Those are the moments that your patients and family members will remember forever. And you are a part of it. It's a humbling experience that you cannot begin to imagine until you go through it yourself.

As mentioned earlier, doctors are customers, too. As with other customers, you'll encounter doctors with different kinds of personality types and communication styles. You will encounter doctors that you really like and respect and others that you would avoid if you could. Some will take an interest in you and explain procedures as they perform them. They'll "go the extra mile" for their patients and express their appreciation for the efforts of their staff. Others may appear smug, dispassionate, or indifferent. They may treat you as if you're invisible or unimportant. One day a doctor will be friendly, and the next day he or she will remain aloof. A doctor may appear quite angry when interacting with you, yet his or her source of anger may have nothing to do with you at all. Sometimes doctors can be demanding and intimidating. Try to keep in mind that doctors are people, too. They have hopes and dreams, feelings and fears, frailties and flaws just like the rest of us. Much of the time they're in a hurry and under a great deal of stress. Some literally hold life and death in their hands on a daily basis. Practicing medicine is an enormous responsibility and it takes its toll. Until you have "walked in their shoes" you have no idea what their lives are like.

Occasionally a doctor may ask you to do something that's outside of your scope of practice. He or she may mistake you for a different type of worker or may not be familiar with your training and job duties. If this happens, speak up! Don't just go ahead and do something you aren't qualified to do because a doctor asked you to. Say politely, "That's not within my scope of practice but I'll go get someone who can help you." If you are competent, diligent, and apply your best communication and customer service skills, you'll likely get along just fine with the doctors.

Guests in your facility are also customers and they, too, are a diverse group of people. Some may be lost or stressed out, running late for an important meeting or a job interview. Others may be in the building to attend a conference or keep an appointment with someone in management. Probably the most frequent request you'll get from guests is help with directions. If you work in a large building, make sure you know your way around so you can give good directions to other people. If you have the time or are headed in that direction anyway, offer to walk with someone to make sure he or she gets to the destination. If someone is waiting to see your supervisor or someone else in your area and you have access to coffee or a soft drink, offer the person a beverage. If someone's pager goes off, direct him or her to the nearest telephone. If you know someone is going to have to wait for awhile, let the person know and explain why. Do whatever you can to make guests comfortable. Your customers will appreciate even a small gesture of kindness.

The last group of customers is vendors. As mentioned previously, vendors are people who work for companies that your company does business with. Vendors might be salespeople from a patient supply or equipment company. They might be insurance agents or drug company representatives. They might work for advertising agencies or temporary services. Just like other customers, they too should be treated with respect and good manners.

There are many factors involved in interpersonal relationships with employees and in providing good customer service. Chapter Four explores how your personal life impacts your professional reputation.

L E A R N I N G   A C T I V I T I E S

Using information from Chapter Three:

❏ Respond to the What If? Scenarios below

❏ Answer the Review Questions below

❏ Watch the video for Chapter Three on the accompanying Student CD-ROM and complete the CD-ROM assignments

What If? Scenarios

Think about what you would do in the following situations and record your answers.

1. Your supervisor has given you a project to complete. There's no way you can possibly get it done, and done well, by yourself in time to meet the deadline. Your coworkers have expressed willingness to help, but you're used to working alone.

2. Three coworkers approach you, angry about a new policy. They're rounding up support to complain to the administration and want you to get involved.

3. A new person joins your work group. She's much older than everyone else and no one seems to like her. It's time to go to lunch and your coworkers leave her behind.

4. At an employee recognition dinner, the head of your company calls you to the stage to praise you for creating a new inventory tracking system. Although three of your coworkers helped you a lot, their names aren't mentioned.

5. Your company offers a six-month, part-time equipment repair course free of charge to employees. Those who enroll attend the classes on paid time. The company also pays the fee for course graduates to become certified as equipment repair technicians. After completing the course and becoming certified, you spot a newspaper advertisement recruiting certified equipment repair technicians for a company that competes with your employer and pays more.

6. You've been on call the last two weekends and it's your turn to be off. At the last minute, a coworker asks if there's any way you could take call for her this weekend. Her brother was seriously injured in a car accident and needs her to help take care of his children for a couple of days. You don't have any plans yourself, but you've already taken call two weekends in a row.

7. A team has been formed to design a new care plan for lung transplant patients. The team's goal is to streamline the process of moving patients from surgery, to a patient care unit, to discharge, and then follow up after they've returned home. Team members include registered nurses, patient care assistants, respiratory therapists, surgical technologists, and home care personnel. Team meetings seem to be going nowhere. Several personalities clash, people disagree on how to get started, and no one listens to each other.

8. One of your coworkers is really beginning to annoy you. He takes longer breaks than he's supposed to and seems to disappear when there's work to be done. This morning, he kept a patient waiting for 20 minutes while he made several personal phone calls. When you remind him he has a patient waiting, he says, "Mind your own business! I'll get to him when I'm ready!"

9. You hear through the grapevine that a coworker has been spreading gossip about you. You're so angry that, as soon as she walks in the room, you're anxious to tell her just what you think of her behavior.

10. One of your coworkers is on corrective action for misspelling several medical terms on patient records. Unless she passes a medical terminology test by the end of the month, her job could be in jeopardy. She's lost her confidence and isn't sure if she can do it.

11. A hospitalized patient has a medical condition that you suffered yourself six months ago but the patient isn't aware of this. He asks if you have any idea what he can expect from his treatment plan.

12. Your teammate finds out that you expressed some doubts about his competence on a recent 360-degree performance appraisal initiated by his supervisor. You value your relationship with him but you're leaving on vacation early tomorrow morning, your teammate has already left work for the day, and you are in a hurry. Sending him an email message from home tonight would be the quickest way to explain your input on his performance appraisal.

Review Questions

Using information from Chapter Three, answer each of the following.

1. Describe the concept of interdependence and list three techniques to strengthen teamwork and interpersonal relationships.

2. Explain why coworkers should be treated as customers.

3. Discuss two ways to demonstrate loyalty to your coworkers and your employer.

4. Identify four types of workplace teams and explain how they differ.

5. Discuss how personality differences can cause conflicts in the workplace.

6. Define *diversity*, list five examples of cultural differences, and explain why it's important to have a diverse health care workforce.

7. Explain the role of respect, good manners, and courtesy in the workplace.

8. Describe why communication skills are the basis for effective relationships.

9. List three problems that may occur when communicating electronically and describe three ways to prevent them from happening.

10. Define *conflict resolution* and explain its importance.

11. List the four styles of communication, identify which is most effective in conflict resolution, and describe the potential impact of each style.

12. List four types of customers found in health care settings and give five examples of good customer service.

13. Describe five ways to provide good customer service for hospitalized patients and their family members.

CD-ROM Assignments

Select Chapter Three on the accompanying Student CD-ROM and complete the assignments.

chapter four

Professionalism and Your Personal Life

"I know the price of success: dedication, hard work, and an unremitting devotion to the things you want to see happen."

Frank Lloyd Wright, Architect, 1867–1959

"How far you go in life depends on your being tender with the young, compassionate with the aged, sympathetic with the striving and tolerant of the weak and strong. Because someday in life you will have been all of these."

George Washington Carver, Agricultural Chemist, 1861–1943

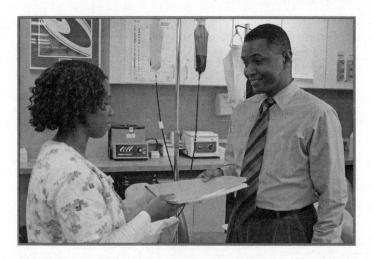

Professionalism in Action

The Student CD-ROM that accompanies this book contains video scenarios and other learning activities related to this chapter. Once you complete reading this chapter, turn to the CD-ROM to gain a richer understanding of the concepts presented here.

Chapter Objectives

Having completed this chapter, you will be able to:

- Define *personal skills* and explain how they affect your success as a health care worker.
- Define *personal image* and describe how your personal image affects the patients you serve.
- List five appearance and grooming factors that result in a professional image.
- Discuss stereotypes and how they impact first impressions.
- List three examples of annoying and troublesome personal habits.
- Describe how grammar and vocabulary impact your professional image.
- Discuss the importance of maintaining professionalism after hours.
- Define *personal management skills* and give three examples.
- Explain the importance of good time management skills and list five techniques to improve them.
- Explain the importance of good personal financial management skills and list five techniques to improve them.
- Explain the importance of good stress management skills and list five techniques to improve them.
- Describe the importance of critical thinking and problem solving skills and list the steps involved in problem solving.
- Identify one challenge unique to your profession and describe how information in this text can help you tackle that challenge.
- Define *adaptive skills* and explain why the ability to manage change is so important in health care today.

Key Terms

adaptive skills	personal skills
critical thinking	practicum
dress code	problem solving
grammar	stereotype
personal financial management	stress management
personal management skills	time management
personal image	well groomed

In previous chapters, we've discussed how professionalism brings together who you are as a person and how you contribute those characteristics in the workplace. We've covered reliability, commitment, character, morals, and how you work with and treat other people. Now it's time to explore the connection between your *personal life* and your *professional life.* Because you're only one person, it stands to reason that if your personal life is out of control, your professional life is going to suffer, too. When you have good **personal skills,** your personal affairs are in order. This frees you up to concentrate on your job and your career. Of course, many of your personal skills transfer to the workplace and influence your reputation as a health care professional. This includes your personal image; your ability to manage time, finances, stress, and change; and your critical thinking and problem solving skills.

What does it take to have a well-orchestrated personal life that puts *you* on the right path to success in your career? Let's examine some personal skills and the impact they have on professionalism and success in the health care workplace.

Personal Image

One of the first things people notice about you is your **personal image**—the total impression you make on other people. Personal image includes your appearance, grooming, and posture; personal habits; and the grammar and language you use. What kind of an impression do you make on people? Are you neat, clean, and **well groomed?** When you come to work, are you dressed properly to perform the duties of your job? Do your appearance and posture convey pride, competence, and professionalism? Do any personal habits detract from your image? How about your **grammar** or the language you use?

Appearance and Grooming

Your personal image is especially important in patient care. Patients need to have confidence in their caregivers. They want assurance that the people caring for them are competent and professional. How would *you* feel if *your* caregiver had a ripped uniform, dirty shoes, oily hair, grimy fingernails, body odor, or bad breath? Would you wonder if that person's unprofessional appearance might also indicate a lack of competence in his or her work?

Other people besides patients are affected by your personal appearance, too. Family members and friends who visit patients also need reassurance that their loved ones are being cared for by professionals. Vendors, guests, and other people who come into your workplace expect to see employees supporting a professional environment. Your coworkers and supervisor expect you to uphold the company's professional standards, too.

Then there's you. When you *look* good, you *feel* good. Setting high standards for your personal appearance not only conveys an image of professionalism to others, it reinforces your pride and self-esteem. How can you expect others to view you as a professional if you don't look like or feel like a professional yourself?

Most employers have a written **dress code** outlining appropriate and inappropriate attire. Sometimes dress code requirements will vary from department to department depending on the duties involved. For example, dietary workers would have a different dress code than departmental secretaries. Be sure you're familiar with the dress code for your job and do your best to uphold it.

Consider the following as a general "rule of thumb." If you don't wear a uniform, select clothing that's appropriate for the duties of your job. Clothes should be clean, pressed, and fit properly. Avoid clothing that is too wrinkled, too frayed, too short, too tight, or too revealing. Shoes should be clean, polished, closed-toe, and worn with socks or stockings. No slippers, flip-flops, or open-toe shoes. Keep makeup, jewelry, and other accessories to a minimum and in good taste. (In some health care professions such as dental assisting, no jewelry is allowed.) Long hair should be pulled back and secured to avoid sanitary or safety problems. Facial hair should be groomed and neatly styled. Avoid wearing perfume or aftershave because aromas may not be welcome among patients and workers and might aggravate breathing difficulties. Poor posture can undermine a professional image. Sit up straight, stand erect, and don't slouch. Make sure to wear your employee identification badge as prescribed in your company's dress code.

Remember, you don't come to work to set new fashion trends or win a beauty contest. Your clothing and accessories should support getting your work done efficiently and safely while instilling a feeling of confidence among those you serve. Save your evening wear, party attire, sportswear, and the latest fashions for after hours. Shorts, capris, leggings, cropped pants, tight pants, tank tops, bare back tops, miniskirts, midriff tops, athletic attire, sweatshirts, sweatpants, T-shirts, painter pants, bib overalls, spaghetti strap dresses, reflective clothing, see-through fabrics, low or revealing necklines, spandex tops and pants, untucked shirttails, and visible undergarments are never acceptable. Even if your employer allows "casual days," remember that you're still in the workplace. If your job involves contact with patients and other customers, avoid wearing blue jeans, T-shirts, or other questionable attire even on casual days. Some employers ban any type of clothing made of denim including scrubs, skirts, shirts, pants, dresses, and jeans regardless of the color. Sunglasses should not be worn unless for medical reasons. The use of head coverings is limited to religious customs or job-specific regulations.

Keep in mind that what constitutes a professional image to one person might be quite different from that which constitutes a professional image to another person. In other words, professional image "is in the eye of the beholder." Such differences often relate to the age and generation of the beholder. Appearance factors that may seem appropriate for your age group may be disturbing to other people, especially those older than you. This includes such things as facial piercing, neon or other non-traditional hair colors, "radical" haircuts and hairstyles, and tattoos. Dress code requirements for health care workers change over time. Many years ago, female nurses had to wear white, starched, uniform dresses with caps on their heads. Have you seen such attire in *any* hospital in recent years? Facial hair on men used to be discouraged. Now, as long as facial hair is groomed, it's rarely an issue. Years ago, women were expected to wear skirts to work because slacks were considered unprofessional. Today, women wearing slacks in the workplace is the norm, especially for those who wear scrubs. In the not-so-distant past, only employees working in surgery were permitted to wear scrubs. In today's hospitals and outpatient settings, it appears the majority of workers wear scrubs. In fact, dress codes for many facilities now not only require wearing scrubs, but also mandate the color and style of the scrubs. (Standardizing scrub colors and the colors and styles of lab coats, shirts, and jackets helps patients and other people differentiate between RNs, LPNs, support staff, and other types of health care professionals.)

Based on history, the dress codes of tomorrow may be significantly different from those of today. But dress codes tend to be conservative, trailing well behind societal trends. Depending on where you work and your job, dress code requirements may limit opportunities for expressing your individuality. You may be expected to dress like everyone else in your department, office, or clinic. You may be subject to a dress code developed by people significantly older than you. As today's younger generation enters the workforce in larger numbers, dress code requirements will change again. Tattoos, body piercing, and so-called radical hairstyles and colors will become more acceptable. Some day, even denim may become the norm! Until then, adherence to current dress codes is a requirement of your job. Always think twice about attire, accessories, or other aspects of personal appearance that might make someone else feel uncomfortable or question your professionalism or competence. Remember that when you are at work, it's all about the patient—not you.

This is a good time to mention the concept of stereotyping. When you are the subject of a **stereotype,** someone has imposed a fixed or conventional mental pattern about you. Stereotypes are often based on appearance and have a major impact on first impressions. When older people see members of the younger generation with facial piercing, tattoos, and non-traditional hairstyles and colors, they may form first impressions based on stereotypes. Such judgments and first impressions are often erroneous but they still occur. Young people may also form first impressions of older people, again based on stereotypes and inaccurate judgments.

Do you form first impressions of other people based on your stereotypes? Do other people form their first impressions of you based on their stereotypes? Most likely, both answers are, "Yes." Stereotyping is a fact of life. But if you remain aware of it, you can counteract its impact. If someone applies a negative stereotype to you based on appearance factors related to your generation, once they get to know you your professional behavior will result in a much more accurate impression. But initially, they may react to you based on their first impression. Some patients may ask to have a "different" health care worker assigned to their care, typically referring to some other worker who would better fit the patient's stereotype of a professional-looking person. It's situations such as this that cause health care employers to establish conservative dress code policies. No health care company wants their patients to be fearful of their caregivers. So dress codes prohibit facial piercing, visible tattoos, and non-traditional hair colors and styles to reduce concerns among patients and visitors.

When interviewing for jobs or working in a health care setting, don't be surprised if people stereotype you based on generation-related appearance factors. Counteract their first impressions with competent, caring, professional behavior and help them get to know you better. Over time, these types of stereotypes may diminish. Try to avoid stereotyping and judging other people yourself and give everyone you meet the benefit of the doubt.

Speaking of stereotyping, one's weight needs to be mentioned briefly. Although it's a sensitive issue, people who are extremely overweight may notice an adverse affect on job opportunities. Although we would like to believe that body weight is not a factor in employment decisions, it happens. Overweight people may be stereotyped as lazy and unable to muster self-discipline. Yet in reality, one's weight may have no bearing on productivity and self-control. The issue of limited space may come into play. A manager may say, "He would not be considered for this job because the space he would have to work in is too cramped and confining for him to function properly." In surgery, there may be concerns about an obese worker contaminating a sterile field in a cramped environment. In radiology, equipment controls may be housed in cubicles too confining for a large person. In jobs requiring heavy lifting or frequent physical activity, employers may feel that such activities could jeopardize the health and safety of an overweight worker. Although it's unfortunate that a person's body weight could have a negative impact on his or her career, it is a fact of life. If you are seriously overweight and wish to do something about it, work closely with your family physician to plan a safe and healthy course of action. If you are content with your weight, or for medical reasons are unable to reduce your weight, be on the lookout for employment opportunities where weight is not a factor.

Personal Habits

Personal habits are also part of your image and sometimes they can be annoying or troublesome to those around you. For example, don't wear noisy shoes or jewelry that jangles. Don't chew gum, pop your knuckles, bite your fingernails, or play childish pranks on coworkers. Avoid eating or drinking in view of patients and visitors. If you have difficulty hearing well, get fitted for a hearing aid. Asking people to repeat everything they say to you can become very annoying. Don't interrupt people when they're talking, and avoid completing sentences for someone else.

In most workplaces today, smoking cigarettes, cigars, and pipes has become taboo because increasing numbers of companies have gone smoke-free. If employees must smoke, they often must do so in designated "smoking huts" or outside the building, huddled together on public sidewalks, presenting a not-so-professional image to the public. Many health care employers now completely ban smoking on their campuses and some won't even allow employees on-site if their clothing emits the odor of smoke. If you must smoke, make sure you're familiar with your company's smoking policies. Confine smoking to designated areas to protect others from secondhand smoke. If your smoke breaks become too frequent or last too long, absence from your work site could become a performance issue. If you smoke and wish to quit, join a support group and get your physician's advice. Many employers now offer free smoking cessation classes for employees. Some employers hire only nonsmokers. Just as being extremely overweight may have an adverse affect on job opportunities, so may smoking. It's hard to maintain your professional image when engulfed in a cloud of smoke or wearing clothing that reeks of cigarettes.

Language and Grammar

The language you use can also reflect personal habits that other people might find annoying. Unless you're talking with your spouse or significant other, don't refer to people has "honey," "sweetie," or "dear." Adult females are "women," not "girls." Adult males are "men," not "boys" or "guys." Some language is totally unacceptable in the workplace, such as obscenities; sexually explicit or risqué comments; and terms that demean members of any racial, cultural, or ethnic group. "Street language" and language that might be acceptable after hours with your family or friends may be viewed as objectionable by coworkers, patients, or visitors. Words such as "fart" and "suck" are becoming more common in public, but are still considered inappropriate in the workplace. Telling jokes in poor taste and making "off-color" remarks is not a good idea even during breaks. Remember the prior discussion about sexual harassment and creating an uncomfortable work environment for others. Even if you mean no harm, someone else's perception might be different. Always be respectful of other people's points of view and avoid using language they might not find appropriate.

Grammar is an important part of your personal and professional image, too. Poor grammar is a warning signal, indicating a lack of education and refinement. Avoid mismatching the subject and verb in a sentence. For example, "We was there" should be "We *were* there." Or, "I seen you do that" should be "I *saw* you do that." "Me and him" should be "He and I." "She don't know" should be "She *doesn't* know." Poor grammar is learned and then reinforced by the people you associate with. It starts with your family as a child and expands to your friends and fellow students. Contemporary music, advertisements, and the media often reinforce poor grammar (i.e., the lyric, "It don't matter to me."). If people close to you use incorrect grammar, it's likely you will too without even realizing it. Just being aware of the need for good grammar might help. If your grammar is weak, work towards improving it. You might be surprised how much it can affect your personal and professional image.

Remember the old saying, "You only get one chance to make a good first impression." You might have only one opportunity to make a favorable impression at a time when it really counts. But, in health care, *every* impression you make is important. As discussed earlier, to patients and other customers, *you* are the company you work for. If you appear unprofessional, so might your company. Put together a total personal package that portrays a professional image. It's a big part of your job and it can make or break your reputation as a professional.

Maintaining Professionalism after Hours

At first glance, you might not realize that, even when you're at home after work hours, some of your actions can affect your professional image. For example, how do you answer your telephone at home? What kind of impression does your recorded telephone message make on people who call you? Don't assume that every caller is a friend, family member, or stranger trying to sell you something. What if your supervisor calls, or a potential employer? Your personal telephone is an extension of your personal image so think about who might be calling you and the impression you want to make on them. Keep in mind that the content you post on the Internet, or that other people post about you, is public information which can positively or negatively impact your professional reputation. Employers are increasingly viewing employee web sites and blogs to search for content that might cause concerns or reflect poorly upon the company. Some employers are putting policies in place which may lead to corrective action or dismissal when employees display an unprofessional image on-line.

Your relationships, both at work and outside of work, can have a positive or negative effect on your personal and professional image, too. The types of people with whom you associate are a reflection of who you are as a person. What impact do the people with whom *you* associate have on your reputation?

It's a small world. You never know when you might run into your supervisor, a coworker, or someone who knows someone you know after hours. "So what?" you might ask. "If I'm not at work, what difference does it make? What I do on my own time is no one's business." While it's true you are "off the clock," what you do after hours can make a great deal of difference. Your reputation goes with you *every place* you go. You never know who might be sitting across the room from you in a restaurant, bar, or some other public place. If you've had a few drinks and your voice gets loud, spreading gossip, revealing confidential information, or criticizing your employer can all come back on you. If you call in sick when you really aren't and then go out in public, you never know whom you might encounter. If someone sees you and word gets back to your supervisor, you wouldn't be the first person to get fired from a job under circumstances like these. If you are arrested and spend the night in jail, don't be surprised if your employer finds out.

If your work group, department, or company has a special event after hours, the standards that govern acceptable behavior at work apply during those events, too. Just because you're with coworkers outside the work setting doesn't mean the rules for professional behavior have changed. Conduct yourself in a professional manner. Don't overdrink, engage in wild behavior, and then regret it the next day. It's hard to reestablish trust, respect, and your professional reputation after making some poor decisions the night before.

Give serious thought to the pros and cons of dating someone you work with before you decide to do it. How might this different type of relationship affect both of you at work? What might happen if and when the relationship ends? Is it possible this person might end up being your boss someday or your subordinate? Avoid social relationships with your boss or with people who report to you. These kinds of relationships can lead to trouble. If things go sour with your boss, you may have to change jobs. If you "mix business with pleasure" with the people who report to you, you may have difficulty supervising them later on.

The point of this discussion is that you are only one person. You aren't one person at work and a different person after work, so do your best to maintain a positive image after hours, too. It's OK to "let your hair down" and have a good time, but don't let your guard down, too. Always think before you act.

Personal Management Skills

Personal management skills help determine how well you manage your personal lifestyle. Having your personal life in order helps support your success at work. Attendance and punctuality are good examples of how your personal life can affect your job. After all, does it really matter how professional you look or how competent you are if you can't get to work on time and be there when you're supposed to be? Your ability to show up for work on a daily basis and keep your appointments are some of the most important aspects of your job. If you have trouble managing your time, handling your finances, dealing with stress, or adapting to change, your personal life could have a negative impact on your job and your career. Let's take a closer look.

Time Management

When it seems like there are never enough hours in the day to get everything done that needs to get done, **time management** skills can be a big help. How well do you manage your time? Do you allow enough travel time to get from one place to another? Do you avoid booking yourself to be in two places at once? Are you sufficiently organized to get things done in a reasonable amount of time? Do you plan ahead for when your car might break down, the bus might be late, or your child or spouse might get sick? How well do you allocate your time to balance work, family, and other priorities in your life? Can you keep things organized at home and still hold down a job? Can you maintain your family and work obligations and still find time to work toward another career goal?

If managing time is a problem for you, here are some suggestions. Use an electronic or pocket-sized calendar to record your class and work schedule and the dates, times, and places of appointments, meetings, family and social activities, and other important events. Refer to your calendar every day and think about what's coming up tomorrow. Allow plenty of time to get from one activity to the next and plan ahead for the unexpected. Always anticipate that things might take longer than you had hoped. If traffic is heavy in the morning, if you might have trouble finding a parking place, or if bad weather could slow you down, schedule some extra travel time to avoid being late. If the public transportation system is unreliable, have a plan for days when the bus is running late. If you ride with someone else, have a plan for when emergencies arise. If you have a personal doctor's appointment, allow some extra time in case the doctor is running late. If you have children, plan ahead for when they get sick or when your babysitter or child care provider is not available at the last minute. Scheduling things too closely together and then encountering unexpected delays can put you behind schedule for the rest of the day.

Don't procrastinate! If something needs to be done, schedule time to do it and get it over with. Letting things build up is a sure way to become overwhelmed and disorganized. Effective organizational skills are vital in time management. Look for ways to become more productive and efficient. If you have a lot of paperwork to manage or records to maintain, have a good filing system so you can put things away and then find them quickly when you need them. Avoid becoming snowed under by huge projects. Break them down into smaller pieces and tackle one step at a time.

Make written lists of things that need to be done, rank each item according to its priority, and then check things off as you complete them. When a task requires concentration, find a quiet place to work that's free of interruptions. Sometimes this might mean going to the public library or working at home after everyone else has gone to sleep. If you become overwhelmed with responsibilities, decide which are the most important and which you can let go. Eliminate activities that waste time and learn to say "no" when you're overbooked.

Most everyone is limited on how much paid sick leave and vacation time he or she gets as part of the job. Wise use of your paid time off is a crucial part of your overall time management strategy. If you use your sick time when you really aren't sick, what will happen if you do get sick and have no paid time off to cover your absence? We've already discussed the fact that professionals don't come to work sick and spread their germs to everyone around them. So if you must stay home to recover from an illness but you've already used up all of your sick time, can you afford to be off work with no pay? And if you're off sick but have no sick time to cover it, could your absence soon become a performance issue that might cost you your job? The best way to avoid these kinds of situations is to use your sick time wisely. Remember—plan ahead and expect the unexpected. Save your sick time for when you really need it and use your vacation time for the other days you want to be off from work. As will soon be discussed, managing your vacation time wisely is important, too.

It goes without saying that your job should be a top priority in your life and in your personal schedule. But your family must be a top priority, too. Always keep in mind what's most important and plan your schedule around your priorities. You can't create more hours in the day, but you can seize control of the time you have. After all, time is one of your most precious and most limited commodities. Learning how to manage it appropriately can have a huge impact on your personal and professional life.

Personal Financial Management

Managing another precious and limited commodity—your personal finances—can also have a major impact on your personal image and on your reputation as a professional. How effective are your **personal financial management** skills? Are your personal finances under control? Do you overspend and rely on credit cards with high interest rates? Do you have trouble paying your bills on time? Are you behind in repaying loans? Is there a chance a creditor might call you or your employer at work or send a tow truck to the parking lot to repossess your car? Could personal financial problems cause you embarrassment at work?

Professionals have their personal finances in order. This doesn't mean they're wealthy—they've just learned to live within their means and practice good financial planning. The following are some helpful suggestions. Develop a budget, monitor and control your expenses, and make the most of your limited financial resources. Read the fine print and familiarize yourself with interest rates and repayment requirements before doing business with companies that offer payday loans, rent-to-own furniture, and tax refund anticipation loans. Keep your checking account balanced and maintain accurate records of how much money you have coming in and going out each month. Match up paydays with the dates you pay your bills to avoid having to pay extra fees because your payments were late.

Delay buying something until you have the money to pay for it. Avoid the temptation to buy things on credit—especially items you don't absolutely need. In most cases, one major credit card should be sufficient. Use that card only for emergencies or to make purchases that you already have the cash to cover. When your monthly bill arrives, pay the balance in full. If you cannot pay the balance in full, make sure your credit card has the lowest interest rate and annual fee available. In addition to paying the interest that's due each month, always pay something to help lower the balance, too. If you're already in debt due to using your credit cards too often, work with a financial counselor to pay off your debts and then *stop* using your cards.

If you possess several credit cards, either discontinue all but one or put the extra cards away someplace where you won't be tempted to use them. If you do decide to keep your extra cards, remember that you may still be subject to annual fees to keep each card current. Excess credit cards may also affect your credit rating because they may be viewed as "potential" debt.

Sound financial planning applies to other kinds of credit purchases too, such as automobile and home loans. Before you buy a car, think about your monthly income and other expenses. How much can you actually afford for a car payment? What about car insurance, license plates, gasoline, maintenance, and parking expenses? When applying for a loan to purchase a home, ask yourself how much you can afford as a house payment each month. What about home insurance, property taxes, and termite inspections? What might happen when your furnace breaks down or the living room carpet needs to be replaced? Millions of Americans have become overwhelmed with credit and loan debts, everyday living expenses, and unexpected repair bills. Serious financial problems can occur quickly and easily, yet it can take years to dig yourself out of a deep financial hole. Thinking about sound financial decisions in advance can keep this from happening to you.

Even if you have little money left after paying your bills each month, it's still important to have a savings plan and to stick with it. A savings account can help you cover unexpected expenses and put some funds away for the future. One of the best ways to save money is through a payroll deduction plan where you work. Money is taken out of your paycheck before you receive it and deposited into an interest-earning savings account. Even if the amount is small, you'll be surprised how quickly the balance can grow. The same is true for investments. A small amount of money deducted from your paycheck and invested wisely can reap significant rewards years from now. Even if you're young, think about investing some money in a retirement fund. These types of investments may be exempt from income tax until you withdraw the money years from now and when you get close to retirement you'll be glad you took the time to plan ahead. The same is true if you're planning to go back to school someday to continue your education or if you must finance the education of your children or other loved ones. College is expensive and it's never too soon to start saving and planning ahead.

Don't forget the need for insurance. How much and what types of insurance are required to protect yourself and your family from accidents and catastrophic events? It's easy to ignore the need for insurance and to spend that money on something else. But if you own a car, a home, or other personal assets, you should protect your investments with an adequate amount of insurance. Consider the need for life insurance and how much health insurance is adequate to protect yourself and your loved ones. If you have insurance benefits at work, make sure you're familiar with them and are using them to the fullest potential. If not, get some counseling from an insurance agent you can trust. Find out if liability insurance is recommended for people who work in your profession. This is especially important for some types of licensed professionals.

Set priorities for how to allocate your limited financial resources and then make your financial decisions accordingly. Sometimes it's better to buy a used car rather than a new car or to buy a smaller home rather than a larger home if the extra money is needed for savings, adequate insurance coverage, or planning for your future. Think twice before loaning money or cosigning for a loan for friends, relatives, or coworkers. Can you get by without that money if the loan is never repaid? If you must loan money, make sure you have a written, signed agreement detailing plans for repayment.

Stress Management

Having to make financial decisions can be a source of stress in your life, but there are many other stress-related factors too, not the least of which is working in health care. In fact, jobs in health care are among the most stress-producing occupations in the United States. Many health care workers function under a great deal of pressure. Jobs may involve lots of responsibility, physical and mental exertion, the need to respond quickly, and the challenge of interacting with diverse groups of people who are under a lot of stress themselves. Effective **stress management** skills can be quite valuable in both your personal life and at work. Your ability to manage stress is also a key factor in your personal image as a professional. If you "blow up," "melt down," or run for the door at the first sign of stress, you may be letting your coworkers and your patients down. Your ability to perform the duties of your job may be affected and your personal health and wellness may suffer. Good stress management techniques can help you keep everything in balance and add more enjoyment to your life.

To manage stress, you must be able to (1) recognize *when* stress is affecting you, (2) understand *how* and *why* stress is affecting you, and (3) identify *where* the stress is coming from before you can take action to alleviate your stress. For example, maybe you felt some stress yesterday afternoon when your supervisor called you into her office. Think back to that situation and examine it more closely. Did you feel stress any other time yesterday afternoon or only when you got called into your supervisor's office? Did you experience that same feeling when she called you into her office last week too, or only yesterday afternoon? Exactly *when* is the stress experienced? Then think about *how* the stress is affecting you. Does it make you feel anxious, nervous, or worried? Do you feel as if something bad is about to happen to you? Then ask yourself *why.* Why does getting called into your supervisor's office cause you to feel stress? What happened the last time you got called in or what did you hear happened to someone else who got called in? Asking yourself questions like these can help you figure out *where* the stress is coming from. Unless you can identify the source of your stress, it can be difficult to deal with it or eliminate the stress altogether. Maybe you made a mistake on a patient's chart, forgot to clock in this morning, or had a disagreement with a coworker. Maybe your supervisor has found out and wants to discuss the matter with you. Or maybe a week ago you got called in because of poor attendance and you know your supervisor has been watching you closely. Getting called into her office again could mean corrective action or getting fired from your job. In any case, the important thing is to know when you're affected by stress, how and why it's affecting you, and where it's coming from so you can decide what to do about the situation. Once you've identified the source of your stress, you can sometimes totally eliminate it. For example, if you know getting called into your supervisor's office can be a stressful situation for you, make sure your attendance, work performance, and interpersonal skills are all good. Then when you get called in the next time, maybe you'll be more optimistic. After all, perhaps your supervisor wants to pass on a letter she received from a patient, acknowledging how much he appreciated the extra kindness you showed him during his last stay at the hospital. Or maybe she wants to invite you to participate on a new committee or help with an upcoming project.

Obviously, there are many other sources of stress besides concerns about your supervisor. Maybe you get stressed out when you have to rush. Would better organizational and time management skills prevent you from having to rush so often? Maybe just the thought of having to get up in front of your coworkers next week to give a report makes you break out in a cold sweat. Would practicing in front of family members or friends first help? Maybe having to take a test for a course you're enrolled in has your stomach tied up in knots. Did you spend enough time studying and preparing for the test? Maybe being verbally attacked by an angry customer increases your blood pressure and makes you want to explode. Would some additional conflict resolution skills help? Just knowing where your stress is coming from can help you decide how to deal with it better.

Not all stress can be anticipated or eliminated and this is especially true when working in the health care environment. You don't always know what's going to happen next and sometimes things can catch you off guard. Maybe a piece of equipment has malfunctioned with no warning, a coworker has called in sick on an unusually busy morning, a new coworker has shown up on your unit with no advance notice, or one of your patients has suddenly gone into cardiac arrest. At times like these, when you're under a great deal of stress, you must stay focused on your job and deal with the situation to the very best of your ability. Then, when the day is over, you need an outlet for your stress. It helps to have someone you can talk with—a person who can relate to what you've experienced and help you think through it. Getting emotional support is especially important for people who work directly with patients. The stress of working with sick and injured people every day can take a toll on the mental health of caregivers. If your job involves this type of stress, or other kinds of stress that wear you down physically, mentally, or emotionally, be sure to seek out professional help when you need it. Your employer may have counselors on staff, chaplains, human resource personnel, or other people who can help when stress becomes too much for you to handle on your own.

Stress can affect your physical health as well as your mental and emotional health. Many physicians and researchers are convinced that stress is a contributing factor to several different diseases and abnormalities. Stress can make you sick and cause symptoms such as headaches, fatigue, sleep problems, diarrhea, indigestion, ulcers, hypertension, dizziness, hives, grinding teeth, skin disorders, and stuttering. Stress has been linked with heart attacks, high blood pressure, alcoholism, depression, and drug abuse. People with "Type A" personalities are among the most susceptible to stress-related disorders. They are highly competitive, impatient, high achievers with strong perfectionist tendencies. They often rush from place to place, work long hours, have an intense drive to get things done, become frustrated easily, and have trouble relaxing. When Type A personalities have a lifestyle that includes smoking, drinking, a poor diet, a lack of exercise, and being overweight, they become targets for stress-related illness. If you're a Type A personality yourself, or if the stress you experience tends to affect your health in any way, don't wait until it's too late. Watch for the warning signs—those personal signals that stress is affecting you—and then seek help in dealing with it.

Stress in your personal life can impact your job, just as stress at work can impact your personal life. Keeping things in balance is the key. Try to keep your stress at work from affecting your home life and your relationships with family and friends. Try to keep stress in your personal life, such as marital problems and financial difficulties, from affecting your work. That's easier said than done because, as has been mentioned previously, you are only one person. Keep in mind that *any change* in your life can be stressful. This includes the death of a spouse or other loved one, divorce, personal injury, or getting fired from your job. Even changes that you perceive as good can produce stress, such as getting married, having a baby, moving into a new home, getting a new job, and graduating from school. Closing on a home mortgage, having a son or daughter move away from home, changing your work schedule, and Christmas can all be stress-producing.

Whenever possible, try to limit the number of stress-producing factors in your life at any given time. For example, try to avoid changing jobs and getting married at the same time, or having a baby and moving into a new home. If you're returning to school while continuing to work, avoid changing jobs if possible or starting a family. The more you can avoid or manage stress-producing factors, the less the likelihood of your suffering any stress-related problems.

Learn to relax and schedule time for recreation, hobbies, sports, and other personal interests. Maintain a healthy balance between work and play. As mentioned earlier, use your vacation time wisely. All workers need time off to rejuvenate themselves and feel refreshed. Get plenty of sleep and exercise, eat properly, and avoid short-term escapes like alcohol and other drugs and smoking. Use your time management skills to help you slow down when you can and stop putting pressure on yourself unnecessarily. Strengthen your interpersonal communication and conflict resolution skills and don't keep negative feelings bottled up inside you.

An important part of managing stress is being happy and well adjusted. Professionals like themselves. They have high levels of self-esteem and self-respect. They have a positive self-image and know they are worthy individuals. It's difficult for others to have confidence in you if you don't have confidence in yourself. Look for the good in yourself. Be patient with yourself and with others. Know your limits and work within them. Avoid being a perfectionist—no one is perfect. Setting unrealistic goals is counterproductive and leads only to disappointment, low self-esteem, and unnecessary stress. Set high but realistic standards for yourself and feel good about your accomplishments.

Strive to enrich yourself. Recognize your potential, learn all you can, and constantly reach for new heights. You have the ability to reach your goals and to excel in your work and your personal life if you learn to manage your stress and not let it rule you.

Problem Solving and Critical Thinking

One of the best stress management tools is good **problem solving** skills. Every day we're faced with a variety of problems to solve, both in our personal lives and at work. By using **critical thinking** skills and a systematic approach to addressing problems, you can usually come up with a solution that will work. You must be able to (1) identify a problem when you see one, (2) define what the problem is, (3) gather information to learn more about the problem, (4) identify possible solutions, and (5) decide which solution is the best.

When faced with a problem, take it one step at a time. What exactly is the problem? It's very important to answer this question before moving on to solutions; otherwise, you might be focusing on the wrong problem. For example, perhaps you've noticed that John, a coworker in your work group, isn't doing his share of the work. It seems as if every time things get busy, John's gone someplace or he's down the hall helping another work group. It's become a problem because his lack of help is slowing things down and preventing you from getting your work done on time. What should you do to solve this problem? Round up your coworkers and everyone confront John? Report him to his supervisor?

First, figure out *exactly* what is the problem. Is John lazy? Does he have an "I don't care" attitude about his job? Does he disappear on purpose, leaving his coworkers to finish up without him? Doesn't he care about his patients? Before you can solve this problem, you need to gather more information. Does John always avoid helping with the work or just at certain times? Is it all types of work he avoids or just certain tasks? When he's gone from his work area, where does he go and what does he do? When he's down the hall with another work group, why is he there and what is he doing? Does it matter if his supervisor is in the area or not?

Upon further investigation, you realize that each time a patient must be moved from his or her bed over to a cart, John is gone from the area. When this happens, you must go find someone else who's available to help lift and move the patient.

Because everyone is busy, it takes at least 15 minutes to round up help and get the patient moved. With several patients having to be moved each day, over the course of your shift you get farther and farther behind in your schedule. Now that you think about it, coworkers are starting to get angry with you because you're pulling them away from their work. The staff in the radiology and physical therapy departments are beginning to complain because your patients are arriving late for their tests and treatments, delaying the schedules in those departments, too. So, if John's not around when it's time to move patients, where is he and what is he doing?

Further investigation shows that John is not just disappearing or lounging in the break room. In fact, he's keeping very busy. He's helping the unit down the hall, rearranging its stockroom to use the same organizational system that your unit just set up. He's also delivering requisitions to the clinical lab and picking up patient charts from the medical records department. He isn't lazy, he doesn't have an "I don't care" attitude about his job, and he does care about patients.

Before long, it becomes obvious that the *only* time John is gone from his work area is when there's a patient to be moved. Having identified the *specific* problem puts you in a much better position to solve it. Instead of accusing John of laziness, reporting him to his supervisor, or labeling him as inconsiderate, you can find out why John disappears when there's a patient to be moved and hopefully work with him to solve the problem. Using your assertive communication skills, you can tell John that his absence during times when patients need to be moved is causing delays. You can tell him you appreciate the fact that he's off helping another unit or doing tasks to help your unit, but when there are patients to be moved, you need help moving them. You've given John the benefit of the doubt, you've explained why his absence is causing problems, and you've done so in a manner that shows your respect for him as a coworker. You may find out that John has hurt his back. He's avoided telling anyone because he knows that lifting and moving patients, equipment, and supplies is part of his job. He might be concerned that, if he can't perform his job adequately, he could get in trouble with his supervisor or even lose his job. So he just disappears at the right time but stays busy still helping out his own unit and other units, too. Now that you know the exact problem and its cause, you and John can work together to solve it.

When faced with a problem, avoid jumping to conclusions. As mentioned earlier, identify and clarify the problem. Gather as much information as you can and then examine the evidence you've found. Decide what options are available to solve the problem and which option would work best. Implement your solution and evaluate the results. In the case of John's disappearance, by using your critical thinking skills and taking a step-by-step approach to the situation, you were able to solve the problem while maintaining a positive relationship with a coworker. There's almost always a good solution to every problem, but you may have to invest some time and energy to find it.

Effective problem solving and critical thinking skills are mandatory for a well-orchestrated personal and professional life. The more you use your critical thinking skills, the better they will get. Working in health care provides lots of opportunities for problem solving, not the least of which is dealing with the many changes that present themselves.

Tackling the Challenges Unique to Your Profession

While the content of this text applies to all health professions, each profession presents some unique challenges based on job responsibilities and customer needs. The more you know about what to expect, the better prepared you will be in applying your critical thinking, problem solving, and other personal skills to tackle these challenges. The table at the end of the Chapter lists examples of challenges faced by some of the many different types of health care professionals. It's important to know what kinds of challenges workers in your profession face and how to be well prepared to meet those challenges.

Managing Change

In today's health care workplace, one of the most important personal skills is the ability to manage change. Just when you think everything is arranged as it should be, something changes. For example, your job might need to be redesigned to fit within a restructured department. You might be given some new responsibilities or be cross-trained to perform some additional functions. You might be reassigned to a different work group or get a new supervisor. Policies and procedures might change, or your work schedule might get adjusted. A new member might join your work team or you might be transferred to a different team. The company you work for might merge with another company or your employer might move to a new location. Your current job might be eliminated.

At the same time you're affected by change at work, you're probably also facing changes in your personal life. Family responsibilities; relationships with friends; and pressures involving finances, housing, transportation, and health all cause many changes over the course of our lives. How well do you deal with change? How effective are your **adaptive skills?** Do you resist change or are you flexible, versatile, and adaptive? It's almost impossible to avoid change. If you are the type of person who resists change, you're going to face some very difficult challenges. On the other hand, if you're flexible, versatile, and adaptive, you're well prepared for the many changes life will throw your way.

Years ago, health care workers were encouraged to learn to *cope* with change. Then, when the pace of change increased, everyone was encouraged to learn to *manage* change. Now, because things change so rapidly in health care, workers must *embrace* change and even *lead* change at times. Successful health care professionals will tell you that change can be a positive influence in your life if you learn to accept it and let it open new doors for you. Having your job redesigned can be pretty scary. You might have to learn some new skills and take on some new responsibilities. But the more new challenges you face, the more you grow. And the more you grow, the better your chances for advancement. View change as positive and learn to make it work *for* you instead of *against* you. After all, do you really want your personal life and your career to be exactly the same five years from now as they are today?

Advancing in your career is a vital part of being a health care professional. Do you have a well-thought-out plan for your future and how you're going to get there? Are you committed to working hard to achieve your goals?

There are two remaining chapters in this book. Chapter Five, "The Practicum Experience," provides information specifically geared for students whose educational programs include a hands-on, **practicum** requirement (i.e., externship, internship, clinicals, etc.). Students in programs with a practicum requirement should read Chapter Five and complete the end-of-chapter learning activities. Even if your educational program does not include a practicum, you will find the content in Chapter Five helpful in preparing for employment. Chapter Six, "Career Planning and Employment," provides valuable information to help when seeking a challenging and rewarding career in health care.

Unique Professionalism Challenges

Professional/Title*	Must be able to:
Administrative Assistant/Secretary	apply strong verbal, written, and electronic communication skills and display exemplary customer service, time management, and organizational abilities
Audiologist	communicate tactfully when patients refuse to acknowledge their loss of hearing and accept the need for hearing aids
Biomedical Technician	perform quickly and accurately under stress when making repairs on urgently-needed patient life support equipment; must devise creative solutions to unusual equipment problems
Cardiac Cath Technologist	perform in a stressful environment, adapting their efforts to the patient's condition and transitioning from diagnostic to therapeutic procedures
Central Service Technician	precisely adhere to sterilization requirements and protocols for preparing surgical instrumentation
Certified Nursing Assistant	withstand the prolonged physical effort of walking, standing, bending, and lifting
Clinical Laboratory Scientist/Technician	perform with accuracy and precision in the collection and processing of specimens and the performance of laboratory tests to ensure that physicians have accurate data on which to base a diagnosis
Dental Assistant/Hygienist	work patiently to educate sometimes reluctant patients about preventative techniques such as proper brushing and flossing and communicate diplomatically when patients ask them to evaluate dental work that was performed by a different dental practice
Dentist	avoid "taking it personally" when patients say, "No offense, but I hate dentists!"
Dietitian	communicate tactfully yet persuasively to convince patients to modify their difficult-to-change eating habits

Echocardiographer — manage stress when scheduling must be ramped up to accommodate ER patients needing to be cleared for cardiac disease to prevent an unnecessary overnight or weekend hospital stay

EKG/ECG Technician

Emergency Medical Technician — undergo cross-training to provide additional functions such as phlebotomy maintain their physical fitness in order to safely move patients awaiting transport to a medical facility

END Technologist — adequately function in a variety of settings including the lab, surgery, and the patients' bedside

Health Information Technician — perform duties with a high degree of accuracy and timeliness and comply with all regulations and laws enacted to protect the confidentiality of patient records and other sensitive information

Licensed Practical Nurse — work within a limited scope of practice and avoid situations where they are asked to perform functions that are legally assigned to registered nurses

Maintenance Personnel — comply with national, state, and local building codes and standards and perform duties with a high degree of safety and vigilance for themselves and those around them

Massage Therapist — apply effective communication skills in promoting the value of massage therapy to a wide range of potential customers and patients

Medical Assistant — master and maintain their competence in both front- and back-office functions even though they may prefer one set of duties over the other

Medical Coder/Coding Specialist — maintain up-to-date knowledge of insurance billing procedures, different coding systems, and annual changes in codes and coding rules

Medical Transcriptionist — ensure hearing and listening acuity and the ability to maintain a high level of concentration for extended periods of time

Nuclear Medicine Technologist — master ever-changing technology (i.e. SPECT/CT, PET/CT, PET/MRI) and fully comply with all radiation safety precautions and regulations

(Continued)

Unique Professionalism Challenges   (Continued)

Professional/Title*	Must be able to:
Nutrition and Food Service Personnel	display effective problem solving and interpersonal skills in interactions with patients, visitors, and staff to resolve dietary and food service issues
Occupational Therapist	demonstrate patience, understanding, and empathy since many patients requiring occupational therapy may encounter lengthy and painful recovery and treatment periods
Paramedic	make quick decisions and initiate treatment without the benefit of physician consultation or knowledge of the patient's complete medical history
Pharmacist	achieve absolute accuracy when the phone is ringing with physician orders, patients are asking questions, technicians are requiring supervision, and patients irate with claim denials are insisting their insurance should cover everything
Pharmacy Technician	earn the respect of a wide variety of people ranging from patients (lay people) to pharmacists to physicians
Phlebotomist	calm patients who are fearful of the sight of blood and needles and who anticipate the discomfort caused by collecting blood samples
Physical Therapist	establish effective therapist-patient relationships within the constraints of limited time, to provide the encouragement and support that patients require during treatment
Physician	actively participate in continuing education to keep up with medical advancements, new pharmaceuticals, research findings, and computerized patient care systems
Physician Assistant	follow protocols to determine when to function independently and when to seek physician consultation
Polysomnographic Technologist	process visual data and utilize decision-making skills to ensure the technical quality of testing data
Psychiatric Technician	utilize effective interpersonal and group dynamics skills to facilitate the development of appropriate social, behavioral, and relationship skills among patients

Radiation Therapist — maintain a daily positive attitude during a four-week treatment period while knowing that about 1/3 of their patients will not survive their disease long-term

Radiographer — demonstrate a strong command of anatomy and computer skills; all diagnostic imaging equipment is moving to the digital realm

Registered Nurse — continually update knowledge and skills to function effectively in a variety of work environments, perform new procedures and operate new medical equipment, and master rapidly-evolving computer software and applications

Respiratory Therapist — apply a diverse array of communication skills to provide patient/family education, converse in very stressful situations such as a code blue, calmly deal with patients who are very ill and unable to breathe, and interact with staff in all areas of the hospital

Sonographer — diagnose medical conditions during ultrasound procedures without disclosing this information to the patient; body language must not reveal what is being seen on the monitor

Speech Pathologist — observe and assess each patient as an individual, to develop a treatment plan that addresses the patient's emotional status, extent of disability, type of disorder, and rate of progress

Support Staff Personnel — apply principles of front-line customer service and follow standards for cleanliness, infection control, and waste disposal to ensure a friendly, safe, and healthy environment for patients, visitors, and staff

Surgical Technologist — apply effective teamwork skills and maintain their concentration while working in a stressful and cold environment and standing in a confined space for long periods of time until relief arrives

(Continued)

Unique Professionalism Challenges   (*Continued*)

Professional/Title*	Must be able to:
Transporter	calm and reassure patients who are undergoing transport to, or from, anxiety-producing situations
Unit Secretary	prioritize activities in a hectic environment where the needs of nursing personnel, physicians, other hospital staff, patients, and visitors all require attention

(*Professions and titles typically include "certified" or "registered" to identify professional credentials, such as "Certified Surgical Technologist" or "Registered Radiographer." Some professions offer more than one option such as "Certified Medical Assistant" and "Registered Medical Assistant.")

L E A R N I N G   A C T I V I T I E S

Using information from Chapter Four:

❏ Respond to the What If? Scenarios below

❏ Answer the Review Questions below

❏ Watch the video for Chapter Four on the accompanying Student CD-ROM and complete the CD-ROM assignments

What If? Scenarios

Think about what you would do in the following situations and record your answers.

1. Your company's dress code allows denim jeans and T-shirts on Fridays for "casual day." Because you've been cross-trained to fill in for the customer service department when it is shorthanded, it's possible you could be asked to work at the information desk in the main lobby with little or no notice.

2. You've spent six months working out at a fitness center and look really good in tight blouses and short skirts. Hopefully, the cute guy who started working in medical records last week will notice you and ask you out.

3. Some of the employees with whom you eat lunch use crude language and at times it can be overheard by other people in your company's cafeteria.

4. The only free time you have to jog on a regular basis is during your lunch break. Your break is long enough to get some good exercise, but you don't have time to take a shower before resuming work.

5. You and a group of coworkers decide to start meeting at a popular bar on Saturday nights to "let your hair down" and have a good time. On the very first night, one person in your group drinks too much and ends up in a fistfight with a stranger seated at the next table. You overhear the bartender calling the police.

6. It seems there are never enough hours in the day for you to get everything done that you want to do. You work full time, participate in two bowling leagues each week, transport your children to their sporting events, volunteer at a local golf course, belong to three different community organizations, and take two courses each semester toward the degree you've been working on. Last week, you were late for work twice, called in sick the day your son's school was closed because of the weather, and had to cancel a dentist appointment at the last minute. You know your job is important but so are your family, friends, and other activities.

7. You just received a pay raise, giving you an extra $25 in each paycheck. Then the telephone rang and you found out you qualified for a new credit card that you hadn't even applied for. With your pay raise and a $5,000 credit limit, you've got the money you need to buy that new home computer and television set your children have been begging you for.

8. For the past month, you've been having headaches and difficulty sleeping at night. You're less patient with your children and have yelled at them several times. Even though you've been eating more than usual, you seem to have very little energy and can't keep up with physical activities. Yesterday, when your supervisor asked you to work overtime, you blew up and said, "No! Why can't somebody else do it? Why does it always have to be me?"

9. Your job is a 20-minute drive from your home and your car is no longer reliable. It has 105,000 miles on it and needs several repairs. Through payroll deductions, you've saved enough money for a year's worth of car insurance and a down payment on a new vehicle, but you aren't sure you can afford the loan payments every month.

10. The company where you work has merged with another company and as a result several departments have been restructured. The job you've had for five years still exists and several new jobs have been created. You qualify to apply for one of the new jobs but, if you get it, you must satisfactorily complete three weeks of training. The pay for the new job is only slightly higher than your current pay. But after a year of work experience in the new job, you'd be eligible for a promotion with even more pay.

Review Questions

Using information from Chapter Four, answer each of the following.

1. Define *personal skills* and explain how they affect your success as a health care worker.

2. Define *personal image* and describe how your personal image affects the patients you serve.

3. List five appearance and grooming factors that result in a professional image.

4. Discuss stereotypes and how they impact first impressions.

5. List three examples of annoying and troublesome personal habits.

6. Describe how grammar and vocabulary impact your professional image.

7. Discuss the importance of maintaining professionalism after hours.

8. Define *personal management skills* and give three examples.

9. Explain the importance of good time management skills and list five techniques to improve them.

10. Explain the importance of good personal financial management skills and list five techniques to improve them.

11. Explain the importance of good stress management skills and list five techniques to improve them.

12. Describe the importance of critical thinking and problem solving skills and list the steps involved in problem solving.

13. Identify one challenge unique to your profession and describe how information in this text can help you tackle that challenge.

14. Define *adaptive skills* and explain why the ability to manage change is so important in health care today.

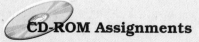 **CD-ROM Assignments**

Select Chapter Four on the accompanying Student CD-ROM and complete the assignments.

chapter five

The Practicum Experience

"Don't waste life in doubts and fears; spend yourself on the work before you, well assured that the right performance of this hour's duties will be the best preparation for the hours and ages that will follow it."

Ralph Waldo Emerson, Essayist and Poet, 1803–1882

"Happiness is when what you think, what you say, and what you do are in harmony."

Mohandas K. Gandhi, Indian Nationalist Leader, 1869–1948

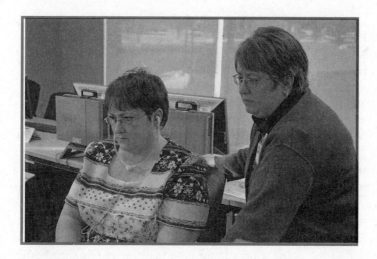

Professionalism in Action

The Student CD-ROM that accompanies this book contains additional learning activities related to this chapter. Once you complete reading this chapter, turn to the CD-ROM to gain a richer understanding of the concepts presented here.

Chapter Objectives

Having completed this chapter, you will be able to:

- Identify the purpose of a practicum.
- List three benefits of a practicum experience.
- Describe three ways to prepare for a practicum.
- Discuss four examples of proper etiquette while on a practicum.
- Describe three ways to ensure success during a practicum.
- Explain the importance of patient confidentiality during a practicum.
- Discuss the value of keeping a journal during a practicum.
- Explain the importance of putting the practicum site first.
- Describe the connection between a practicum and employment after graduation.
- Identify four general policies, procedures, and issues related to a successful practicum experience.

Key Terms

etiquette	profane
journal	penmanship
observations	samples room
office politics	

The Purpose of a Practicum

Educational programs use different terms such as clinicals, externship, internship, hands-on experience, on-site learning, experiential learning, and so forth. But these terms all mean basically the same thing—a "real-life" learning experience obtained through working on-site in a health care facility while still enrolled as a student. For the purpose of this chapter, we refer to all of these as a practicum. Whether you are in medical assisting, surgical technology, radiography, medical technology, or any one of a number of different types of health care educational programs, there's a good chance you'll be doing a practicum-type learning experience before you graduate. Some programs begin the practicum experience early in the curriculum, integrating classroom instruction with hands-on experience. Other programs complete classroom instruction first and schedule the practicum at the end of the program just prior to graduation.

The CD-ROM segments that you viewed during the first four chapters take place in a physician practice but the information presented applies in most health care settings. You may see some of these "real-life" examples during your practicum experience.

The Benefits of a Practicum Experience

Students often ask, "Why should I worry about my practicum? It's just another assignment from my instructor." In reality, your practicum is *much more* than just another assignment. It's one of the most, if not *the* most important part of your education. Your practicum is an opportunity to apply the knowledge and skills you've acquired during the classroom portion of your training in an actual health care setting while still a student. If you perform well, your practicum could also result in an employment recommendation or a job offer when you graduate.

Some practicums include monetary compensation, but most do not. It depends on the profession you're in and the educational program you attend. The site supervisor will assign your work hours, break times, duties, and responsibilities. At times you may feel like "free labor." But keep one very important fact in mind—you are there as a *student* to learn and to hone your knowledge and skills. You are *not* there as an employee. Participating in a practicum is a privilege. Whether your practicum is in a physician practice, surgery department, imaging center, or clinical lab, you are a guest in that facility. The site supervisor has the right to terminate your practicum at any point in time if he or she believes that your appearance, attitude, or performance negatively affects the site's patients, visitors, physicians, or employees. So this is an excellent opportunity to "prove yourself." Apply everything you've learned and begin establishing your own reputation as a health care professional.

There's another valuable benefit of doing a practicum. It may help you determine what types of patients you'd like to work with after graduation. It's not unusual to hear students say they want to work in pediatrics (peds). Working in peds can be very rewarding, but it takes a certain type of person to do this. Sometimes students have an unrealistic image of working with children. They imagine themselves holding and cuddling newborns and small children. They don't always think about children being sick and parents being upset. Experience shows about half of the students who say they want to work in peds change their minds after a pediatric practicum. Radiography students who think they want to specialize in neuro procedures, or surgical technology students who think they want to scrub in on cardiovascular cases, may change their minds after working with these types of patients during clinicals.

The same may be true for different employment locations. Pharmacy technician students may think that a hospital pharmacy would be their first choice and physical therapy assistants may plan on working in an outpatient rehabilitation center after graduation. But after their practicum experience, the pharmacy techs might instead aim for jobs in retail pharmacies and the physical therapy assistants might seek employment in acute care hospitals. There's nothing like "being there" to know for sure where you'd like to work and the types of patients and procedures you'd like to be involved with. Your practicum can help you make those decisions *before* you accept a job offer, without having to realize later that it's not a good match for you and your career goals.

Your performance during your practicum will be evaluated based on criteria established by your educational program. It's likely that you will receive a grade based on your performance. And, as mentioned earlier, your performance could result in a job offer at graduation. While you are on your practicum, feel free to ask questions. The employees who work there will know that you are a student. They expect you to be a little bit nervous at first and won't hold you accountable for knowing everything when you start. By asking questions, you will show an interest in what goes on at the site. While it's a good idea to ask questions, it's equally important to remember the answers and not ask the same questions repeatedly. Asking the same questions multiple times could not only irritate people, it could make you appear incompetent. If you want to remember something important, write it down on a notepad. (The value of the notepad will be discussed later in this chapter.)

Picture a large medical office where two students are doing their practicum at the same time. One student is always visible, asking questions and taking notes. The other student is always off someplace else, socializing or taking a smoke break. She rarely asks questions, doesn't show much initiative, and always has some reason why she has to leave early every week. Surely it's obvious which student will receive the highest grade. What neither student knew was that there was going to be a position opening up about the same time the practicum ended. In this case, the practicum was not "just another assignment" but was actually a multiweek job interview.

Preparing for Your Practicum

Depending on your educational program, you may be assigned to a practicum site or you may have some choices. If you have choices, there are some important things to take into consideration before making your decision. It is recommended that you *do not* do your practicum at a site where you or your family members are patients as most physicians will discourage this. Some educational programs schedule on-site **observations** for students to visit potential sites prior to selecting, or being assigned to, a practicum location. If you have the option of choosing a practicum site and doing one or more on-site observations first, you should take advantage of this opportunity. During an observation, you'll gain valuable information about the people who work there and the pace at which they work. Is it a friendly, service-oriented facility? How do the employees interact with their coworkers, patients, physicians, and visitors? Is the environment fast-paced or slow-paced? Which type of environment would be most comfortable for you? Some students prefer a fast-paced environment and they get bored when things move too slowly. Other students prefer a slower pace and feel rushed if things move too quickly.

Regardless of whether you're assigned to a site or have some choices, it's a good idea to do some research before you get there. Do they have a web site or printed materials that you could review? The more that you know about the site, the better prepared you will be and the more at ease you will feel on your first day. To prepare for your practicum, "scope out" the site ahead of time and make contact with the site supervisor before your first assigned day. Check with your instructor first to get permission. Then call the site and introduce yourself. Ask about the dress code, even if your instructor has already told you about it. Confirm your start date and the hours that you will be there. If there are days when you will need to leave early for a prior commitment, this is the time to let the site supervisor know. By doing this ahead of time, you will demonstrate professionalism and an interest in the site even before you arrive. Travel to the site a few days before your practicum starts. Note the travel time. What time do you need to leave home in the morning to arrive at your site on time? How much traffic should you anticipate? What if the parking lot is full? What if your bus connection is running late? Imagine the "worst case scenario" and have a contingency plan.

On your first assigned day allow sufficient travel time to arrive at the site at least 15 minutes early so you will feel more comfortable and less rushed. You don't want to arrive late or appear unprepared. Remember, you *never* get a second chance to make a good first impression.

During Your Practicum

Keep a small notepad with you and take notes. Write down questions that you may want to ask later on. When you think of a question, it may not be the appropriate time to ask it. For example, maybe you have a question about the way the physician performed a certain patient procedure. It would be inappropriate to ask in front of the patient because doing so could make the patient (and the physician) uncomfortable. You may have questions that you will want to hold on to until you meet with your program instructor again. During the course of a week, many things will happen and your notepad will really come in handy.

Consider keeping a **journal.** A journal is a private record of your thoughts and experiences. Some educational programs require that you keep a journal to include certain types of information. Your program may be required to keep a copy of your journal in your student file. In such cases, it is best to record your personal thoughts and emotions in a separate document or notepad. To protect patient confidentiality, you should not mention patient names in your journal. Take a few minutes at the end of each day to record what happened, how you reacted, how you felt about it, and whether you could have handled it differently or better. Journaling can help you "re-group" your feelings, process your experiences, and reflect upon what you've learned. Write about both the good and bad things that you see and experience. Record both the things you *do* and *do not* want to do again in the future. Sometimes you may hear an employee being impolite to a patient. Write down what you heard to remind yourself how others may perceive the things that you say. You will likely see some things being done in a different way than the way you were taught.

By recording it, you will remember to discuss this with your instructor and class-mates later on. Expect to be nervous and busy at the same time. If you don't write things down, you may forget some important things. If it's written in your journal, you will have it as a reference whenever you need it. There are also some good pocket-sized reference books for different professions. Check with your instructor to find out if such a book might be helpful during your practicum.

Your site will have policies and procedures outlining what you may, and may not, do as a student. Familiarize yourself with these at the beginning of your practicum and be sure to comply with them. Depending on the profession and site, this may include getting permission from each patient before you are allowed to observe or participate in a procedure. Some patients are comfortable with the idea of having a student present whereas others are not. As mentioned in Chapter One, patients have rights. As a student on practicum you also have rights, including the right to observe and participate in procedures related to your educational experi-ence. But the patient always comes first. If a female patient, for example, is not comfortable having a male student in the room during her procedure, the male stu-dent will typically be expected to comply with the patient's wishes. In most situa-tions, there will be a sufficient number of other patients who are willing to allow student involvement to ensure that educational goals can be met. Make sure you know how your practicum site protects the rights of its patients and comply with those policies and procedures.

Maintaining confidentiality and adhering to HIPAA rules are top priorities. While on your practicum you may have access to patient charts and other private information. You may even know some of the patients. (This is why it's a good idea to *not* do your practicum at your or your family's personal physician's office.) What you see, hear, or read at the site *must* stay at the site. Never read patient charts unless instructed to do so. You will undoubtedly see and do things that you will want to tell your family and friends about, such as unusual cases, certain procedures, and your opportunities to be directly involved. It's natural to be excited and want to share your experiences. But you must remember to never use the patient's name or pro-vide any other descriptive information that could reveal the patient's identity. Here's an example of an acceptable comment:

> You won't believe what I did today. We removed a mole from a patient's arm. I got to prepare the patient for the minor surgery and assist the doctor with the procedure.

You described what you did without breaking confidentiality. Usually while on your practicum, there will be times when you, your classmates, and instructor meet to dis-cuss what you have seen and done during the week. Again, this is a time to protect the confidentiality of the site's patients.

In addition to medical records, you may also have access to other information such as patient financial records or the site's patient charges or financial transactions.

This is information that will need to stay at the site and you should not talk about it. Private information is shared only on a "need to know" basis. That means the information is made available only to those people who need to know it to care for patients and conduct the site's business. You may be rotating to different sites during your practicum, working in companies that compete with one another. Maintain the privacy of business-related information and use discretion when making comparisons among the different places you work. Remember what was said earlier— you are a guest at the site and the supervisor has the right to terminate your practicum at any point should your performance pose a problem. Violation of confidentiality or the unauthorized sharing of sensitive information is a legitimate reason for immediate termination. If you are terminated from your practicum site, you might find it difficult to gain access to another site and your quest for recognition as a health care professional will suffer a major setback.

Many sites have what's called a **samples room.** This is a place (sometimes a closet) where they keep samples of drugs and medical supplies. You may be asked to go there and get samples of something for a patient. Just because the sales reps leave samples at the site at no charge, and the site gives samples to patients at no charge, that does not mean that you can help yourself to anything that you want out of the sample room at no charge. Remember the student mentioned earlier who did not get the job? One of the places to which she was disappearing was the sample closet. This drew attention her way, but not in a good way.

No discussion about proper **etiquette** while on a practicum would be complete without talking about **office politics** and how to avoid them. As you are probably aware, all workplaces have office politics. Whether you're doing your practicum in a physician practice, long-term care facility, or hospital critical care unit, there will be coworkers who don't get along with one another. Sometimes one coworker will tell you something negative about another coworker or complain to you about another coworker to try to get you "on his or her side." This happens frequently with students. You need to stay neutral and not get involved. As time goes by, you may even agree with the coworker's complaints. Should you join him or her in voicing those complaints? Absolutely not. This is one of the biggest problems students face. You are *not an employee* of that site and you may not have all the facts. Some employees will manage to get a student in the middle of a disagreement among coworkers. The student then takes the group's complaint to the supervisor. When the supervisor questions the employees, they deny any involvement. If you were the supervisor, what would you think of the student?

If you allow yourself to become involved in office politics, you may be labeled a troublemaker. The site supervisor may reconsider allowing you to remain there. You could be terminated from the site or lose your opportunity for a good employment reference or job offer at graduation. There's more to a practicum than just practicing your hands-on skills. Practicing your "people skills" and your "professionalism skills" are equally important in ensuring success.

One of the reasons sites agree to allow students to do practicums there is that having a student present keeps the staff "on their toes." Students tend to be inquisitive and ask lots of questions. They watch how coworkers interact with one another and with patients, visitors, and physicians. The employees at the site are all aware of this. They must be able to explain things, answer questions, and set a good example. This helps keep the employees focused on the correct way to do things and cautious about how they interact with, and respond to, patients and one another.

Keep in mind that there's more than one *right way* to do things and *your* way might not be the *only* right way. For example, when you clean a room, do you dust first or vacuum first? Which way is right? Both ways. There are different ways to get the same result. If you see a site employee doing something in a way that's different from the way you've been taught, don't say, "That's wrong" or "You aren't doing that right" or "That is not the way we were taught." Instead, turn it into a learning situation. Ask the person to explain how and why he or she did it that way. You might learn a new technique that's easier or more efficient.

You will likely see different equipment used in your practicum site than what was used in your classroom or laboratory at school. This is one of the benefits of doing a practicum. You get to experience different technology before starting your first job. You should approach this situation by saying, "This machine is different from the one I was taught on. Would you please show me how this one works?" This sounds much better than saying, "I don't know how to work this EKG machine. We were never shown how to do it." With the first example, you are indicating that you know the correct procedure but are not familiar with the equipment. Medical equipment can be complicated to operate. Mistakes can be expensive and jeopardize patient care. The purpose of your being at the site is to learn and gain experience. By making sure you know the correct way to use each piece of equipment, you are demonstrating the importance of putting the site and its patients first.

Once you have learned what is expected of you and you feel comfortable with the equipment and procedures, it's important to begin functioning with less direct supervision. If you are uncertain about something, by all means ask! But if you've been given a responsibility and it's "your job" to do it, then do it. For example, once a patient has checked in and the chart is ready, if it's your job to escort the patient to the exam room and take their vitals, then that's what you should do without waiting to be told. Do not make the patient wait. If you hear the phone ring and you've been instructed how to answer it, then answer it. The more you can do the better. The more you learn to do and the more cross-training you undergo, the more marketable you will become. Keep one thing in mind. You are there to learn and to help, not to stand around and get in the way. Show initiative. One of the quickest ways to be labeled as unprofessional is to stand around doing nothing. Everyone from the receptionist to physicians will be watching your every move. Avoid spending too much time chatting with the staff. Be productive and help keep the site moving smoothly.

Here's a story that actually happened in a large medical office. A medical assisting student reported to the office on her first day. When she arrived, she could not remember the name of her contact person. As she was talking to the person seated at the receptionist desk, she became discouraged and used some **profane** language. As it turned out, the "receptionist" was actually the office manager who was in charge of hiring for the practice. You can use your imagination as to how the student's practicum assignment went and whether or not she was offered a job there at graduation.

Unprofessional language should never be used in your practicum site. That is not to say that you won't hear it yourself because you will. But just because you hear the employees using profane language is no excuse to use it yourself. Put yourself in the patients' position. If you were sitting in the waiting room and heard the staff using profanity, how would you feel? What impact would it have on your opinion of the company? Would it become a factor in deciding whether or not to continue going there for your health care or recommending the company to other people? What if you were a new patient and this was your first visit? At each step of the way, put yourself in the patients' shoes. Remember that, even though you are there as a student, the patients will consider you part of the staff. Your behavior not only affects your own reputation but that of the site. Using profanity or any other type of unprofessional language will undermine both reputations.

In Chapter Three, cliques were discussed. While on your practicum, you should avoid becoming part of a clique. Depending on how long you are there, you may start to feel comfortable with the staff and feel as if you "belong." Belonging is a good feeling, but there's a difference between "fitting in" and being part of a clique. Fitting in simply means that you work well with the staff and are seen as cooperative. Your personality may blend well with the personalities of the employees. Being part of a clique, however, can work against you. Cliques are groups of people who stick together and don't really associate with the rest of the staff. They're exclusionary and they impede effective teamwork. Often, employees in cliques are less productive because they spend too much time socializing and gossiping. Supporting teamwork should be one of your goals. When everyone works well together, the site functions as a "well-oiled machine." During your practicum, pay attention to which employees are good team players. Note the difference between team players and nonteam players. You'll notice that nonteam players have to work harder to get the work done while team players pitch in and help each other out. Strive to be a team player and avoid cliques. This could become a major factor in getting a positive employment reference or a job offer at the end of your practicum.

There are several other things to consider during your practicum. Protect yourself and others from communicable diseases. We all want to "make a difference" in peoples' lives by working in health care. But some people are so scared about catching a communicable disease that they have a difficult time doing their job appropriately. As you participate in your practicum, remember everything you've been taught about how to protect yourself and others. Make sure that you are using protective devices and using them correctly. Some sites will exclude you if you don't use Universal Precautions. Remember, if you don't have enough respect to protect yourself, then you won't have enough respect to protect your patients and/or coworkers. If you become ill during your practicum, don't report for duty and spread your germs to the patients and staff.

While on your practicum, you may come in contact with patients who are familiar with the staff and not at all comfortable with "new" people, including students. Don't take this personally—it's very common. Some patients will refuse to tell the student (or a new employee) anything. The student tries to obtain the patient's history and asks why the patient is there to see the doctor. But the patient just keeps asking for "her nurse." Patients can become very attached to the members of their health care team and reject the involvement of other people. If this happens to you, do not argue with the patient. Explain who you are and why you are there. If the patient still insists on interacting with someone they know, simply excuse yourself and go get one of the staff.

When you walk through the door at your site in the morning, leave your personal problems outside. If you had a disagreement with your spouse or your child that morning, do not discuss it with the people working at your site. If you are upset, distracted, and not thinking clearly, mistakes can happen. In the medical field, there is no room for mistakes.

Never discuss your personal life or your own medical history with patients. You are there to focus on the patient's situation, not your own. The medical profession is a relatively "small world." People who work for one company often know their counterparts at other companies. They participate in the same professional associations and attend the same continuing education conferences. When they get together, it's not uncommon for them to discuss personnel issues. If you're doing your practicum at a site where you *don't* want to work after graduation, just keep in mind that the people who work at that site may well know their counterparts at the site where you *do* want to work after graduation. Your performance and reputation as a student can easily spread from one place to the next without you even knowing about it.

Ensuring Success on Your Practicum

Several factors have been discussed regarding what you need to consider in preparing for and participating in your practicum experience. Achieving success, especially during a lengthy practicum, is not easy. Working without pay can become frustrating and tiresome, especially when you're a student with bills to pay and family obligations to meet. If your practicum occurs at the end of your educational program, you are probably counting the days until graduation and your first paycheck.

If you look at most employment ads, you'll notice that employers seek applicants who have experience. Once you've finished your practicum, you will have experience.

You'll know how the "real world" operates. You'll have firsthand knowledge and insights to share during job interviews. You'll be more polished in your communication skills. And you'll present yourself in a professional manner. You received no pay for your practicum, but the experience you gained is priceless.

Make sure you list the experience you gained during your practicum on your résumé. Ask your site supervisor if you may use him or her as a reference. If you've had a positive experience, most supervisors will be happy to assist you in finding a good job. If you show up on time, avoid unnecessary absences, and do your best to fulfill the goals of your practicum, and all *without pay,* then your supervisor will assume that you will work just as hard, or even harder, for pay.

If you secure a job prior to graduation, and especially if you're hired by your practicum site, don't make the mistake of slacking off just because you "landed the job." Too many students have made this mistake. Once they have a job, they start coming in a few minutes later or taking a longer lunch break. This indicates that they were only trying to make a good impression to get a job. Remember that any job you already have becomes the reference for the next job you seek!

As mentioned earlier, it's likely that you will be receiving a grade for your practicum. When you use your practicum site supervisor as a reference, he or she will be contacted by employers and asked a series of questions about you and your performance. Whether it's assigning a grade or providing an employment reference, similar criteria will be considered when describing your performance. What follows is a list of the criteria that you can expect.

1. Were you dependable?

   Did you show up on time and ready to work? How many absences did you have? If you were absent, did you follow procedures for reporting your absence? No matter how competent you are, if you aren't there you are not doing your job. Employers would rather have a less experienced employee with a good attendance record than an experienced employee with a poor attendance record.

2. Was your appearance professional?

   Were you neat and clean and dressed appropriately? Did your appearance reflect a positive image to your patients and coworkers? Avoid trendy clothing and appearance. You may think that hair streaked in purple is fashionable, but it's not appropriate in a business setting. If you wear jewelry, make sure it's conducive to the work you're doing. Safety comes first when working with body fluids, equipment, and patients. Keep in mind that some professions don't allow any jewelry to be worn for this reason.

3. Did you display a friendly personality and good customer service?

   Did you get along well with patients, physicians, and coworkers? Were you cooperative with the staff and a team player?

4. How well did you work under stress?

   Did you maintain a calm demeanor and balance your priorities appropriately? Did you adapt well to change?

5. How well did you perform your duties with limited supervision?

   Did you demonstrate initiative or wait to be told what to do? Did you accept responsibility and perform your duties competently?

6. Did you display a positive attitude and a desire to learn?

   Were you motivated? Did you ask good questions? Were you eager to learn new procedures and practice what you learned?

7. Did you display a professional image?

   Did you apply everything that's been discussed in this book and on the CD-ROM to make the very best impression you could possibly make?

If you can answer "yes" to all of these questions, you are well on your way to achieving a good grade, a positive employment reference, and recognition as a health care professional.

After Your Practicum

On your last day it's always a good idea to thank everyone at your site. Let them know how much you appreciate the time they allowed you to be there and all of the help and encouragement they provided. Within a few days (no longer than a week) of leaving, send them a Thank You note. When the site receives a Thank You note from a student, it demonstrates initiative, appreciation, and courtesy. When writing the note, make sure you use good grammar and **penmanship.** Thank You notes can become the deciding factor on who gets a job among different applicants.

In Summary

Here are some practicum Do's and Don'ts to keep in mind.
   Do:

- Scope out the site before the first day
- Research the site to learn as much as you can about it in advance
- Keep a notepad with you to write things down
- Remember that you are a guest, not an employee
- Arrive on time and avoid unnecessary absences
- Ask questions and remember the answers
- Dress appropriately
- Put the site and its patients first

- Be respectful
- Show initiative
- Acknowledge that there are other ways of doing things
- Keep a journal
- Protect patient confidentiality
- Adhere to HIPAA regulations
- Display a positive attitude
- Send a Thank You note

Don't:

- Use profane language
- Become part of a clique
- Judge the staff or their way of doing things
- Bring your personal problems to work
- Take excessive breaks
- Ask the same question over and over
- Participate in office politics
- Tell the staff that they are "doing it wrong"

Chapter Six discusses how to pull together everything that you have learned so far to plan an exciting career, secure a rewarding job, and achieve your goals as a health care professional.

L E A R N I N G   A C T I V I T I E S

Using information from Chapter Five:

- ❏ Respond to the What If? Scenarios below
- ❏ Answer the Review Questions below
- ❏ Watch the video for Chapter Five on the accompanying Student CD-ROM and complete the CD-ROM assignments

What If? Scenarios

Think about what you would do in the following situations and record your answers.

1. While escorting a patient to the exam room, she asks you if her husband's tests results are back yet. You know that the results are back, but you don't have permission to give the results to anyone except the patient himself.

2. You notice the constant ringing of telephones in the office. You notice that the receptionist is talking on the telephone. But several times during the day, she's involved in personal calls. In the meantime, the ringing telephones are ignored.

3. One of your patients is a friend of your mother. She's at the doctor's office to find out if she's pregnant. After she leaves, her pregnancy test results come back as negative. You've been unable to reach her by telephone to give her the results. The next day you see her at the mall with her family.

4. You realize that your neighbor is a patient at your practicum site. You see her chart and are wondering why she always looks so tired all of the time. The chart is right there and no one is watching.

5. During your practicum, a patient mentions that he would prefer that no one other than his physician be in the room during his medical procedure. It's a procedure you've never seen before and you would like to observe. The patient will be under the influence of medication and probably won't remember what happened during the procedure.

6. You're short on money and need some antibiotics for your child. Her prescription has run out but there is a large supply of the same drug in your site's sample room. You notice that samples are given to patients free of charge.

7. While on your practicum, you notice that an employee has left work 15 minutes early every day for the past week. Two other employees who suspect this behavior but have not witnessed it themselves ask you to report it to the site supervisor.

Review Questions

Using information from Chapter Five, answer each of the following.

1. Identify the purpose of a practicum.

2. List three benefits of a practicum experience.

3. Describe three ways to prepare for a practicum.

4. Discuss four examples of proper etiquette while on a practicum.

5. Describe three ways to ensure success during a practicum.

6. Explain the importance of patient confidentiality during a practicum.

7. Discuss the value of keeping a journal during a practicum.

8. Explain the importance of putting the practicum site first.

9. Describe the connection between a practicum and employment after graduation.

10. Identify four general policies, procedures, and issues related to a successful practicum experience.

CD-ROM Assignments

Select Chapter Five on the accompanying Student CD-ROM and complete the assignments.

chapter six

Career Planning and Employment

"Give me a stock clerk with a goal and I'll give you a man who will make history. Give me a man with no goals and I'll give you a stock clerk."

J.C. Penney, Retailer, 1875–1971

"My mother said to me, 'If you become a soldier, you'll be a general; if you become a monk, you'll end up as the Pope.' Instead, I became a painter and wound up as Picasso."

Pablo Picasso, Artist, 1881–1973

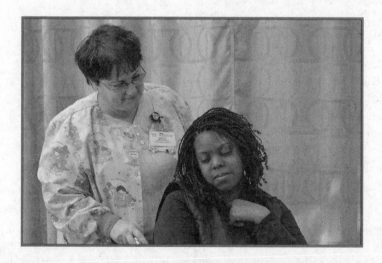

Professionalism in Action

The Student CD-ROM that accompanies this book contains video scenarios and other learning activities related to this chapter. Once you complete reading this chapter, turn to the CD-ROM to gain a richer understanding of the concepts presented here.

Chapter Objectives

Having completed this chapter, you will be able to:

- Explain the difference between a stagnant career and a dynamic career.
- List five questions to ask yourself in career planning and identify three helpful resources.
- Describe personal assessments and what you can learn from them.
- List four ways to explore employment opportunities where you live.
- Define *goals, short-term goals, long-term goals,* and *realistic goals* and explain why goals are important.
- Describe role models and mentors and explain their value.
- Identify the importance of computer skills in career advancement.
- Explain the importance of job application forms and identify four factors in completing them appropriately.
- Describe the role of pre-employment assessments.
- List five important factors in participating in a job interview.
- Describe why continuing education is important for health care workers and list two ways to obtain continuing education.

Key Terms

basic skills

constructive criticism

dynamic

job shadowing

mentors

networking

occupational preferences

official transcript

personal assessments

postsecondary

potential

role models

transferable skills

As mentioned previously, it's important to keep an eye on where your career is headed and to make good decisions about your future. Health care professionals rarely stay stagnant. They're always looking for opportunities to learn new things, acquire new skills, accept new responsibilities, and grow personally and professionally. How much of your **potential** for growth and development has yet to be tapped? What plan do you have for your career post-graduation?

Planning for your future, setting realistic goals, and hanging in there without giving up are important steps in a **dynamic** ever-changing health career. Regardless of your age, don't hesitate to dream and always ask yourself, "What comes next in my professional and personal life?" Although it's important to always keep an eye on where you're headed, don't forget to enjoy "the here and now," too. Remember the saying—life is a journey, not a destination. It's the adventure along the way that makes life worth living. *Plan* for tomorrow, but *live* for today. Stop to "smell the roses" each step of the way. Recognize your accomplishments, celebrate them, and then move on to the next step in your career.

Career Planning

Have you decided what to do when you graduate from school? Have you identified some specific job opportunities and places of employment that appeal to you? Consider your **occupational preferences.** What type of environment do you wish to work in? Do you prefer a large, medium-sized, or small organization? An urban, rural, or small town setting? Do you want to work in the same town where you live now or are you thinking of relocating? If so, what part of your state, or the country, is attractive to you? Do you want to remain in one place or travel from place to place as a "temporary" or "seasonal" worker? Is it important for you to work in a place with the latest technology and medical procedures? Have you thought about access to continuing education and career advancement opportunities? What shift or schedule would best fit your lifestyle, family responsibilities, and personal interests? What types of specific job responsibilities are you seeking? Are you planning to specialize or does cross-training and variety appeal to you? What types of patients, physicians, and coworkers do you wish to work with?

Are you planning to remain in the same job or discipline indefinitely, or do you think you might gain some work experience for a few years and then try something a little different later on? Is a leadership position (supervision, management, administration) part of your plan? Maybe medical research, equipment sales, or education? Although it's important to know what you want to do right after graduation, it's never too early to start thinking about your future. Where you see yourself five years from now should be taken into consideration when deciding what to do first.

Expect to change jobs several times during your career. You may decide to stay in the same health care discipline but apply your knowledge and skills with a different patient population or in a different type of employment setting. Or, you may end up switching to an entirely different occupation as you gain experience and your interests change. One of the many advantages of working in health care is that there are so many different options from which to choose. Sometimes the choices seem overwhelming.

One of the best ways to help make decisions is **job shadowing** to see firsthand what other jobs are like. Learning about employment opportunities in school and reading about jobs and places of employment in newspapers and on web sites can provide valuable information. But there's no substitute for actually *being there* and seeing firsthand what it's like. Make an appointment to meet with people working in the types of jobs and places of employment that appeal to you. Spend some time talking with people and observe the work they do and the environments in which they work. Find out what a typical day is like. Ask people what they like most, and least, about their jobs. What advice might they offer you? If they had it to do over again, would they have made the same decisions?

Another advantage of working in health care is having so many options to apply **transferable skills.** You can change jobs several times and still stay in the same discipline, often working for the same organization. You might want to stay in the same discipline (nursing, medical assisting, surgical technology, radiography, etc.) but progress to a leadership role (charge nurse, office manager, chief technologist, etc.). You might want to make a lateral move into another discipline where your transferable skills can give you a head start (medical assistant to medical coding, etc.). You might want to start as a diagnostic radiographer and then cross-train into sonography, nuclear medicine technology, or mammography. You might decide to return to school in a few years to earn an advanced degree or acquire an additional professional certification. So many choices and so many decisions!

Each step in career planning involves identifying, narrowing down, and selecting options. Expect to do this several times during your professional life. You'll likely be asking yourself, "What do I want to be when I grow up?" more than once! You'll need to reevaluate: (1) your occupational preferences (the kinds of work and work settings you prefer), (2) your abilities and aptitude (your current knowledge and skills, plus your capacity to learn more), and (3) the employment opportunities available to you (access to well-paying jobs with opportunities for advancement near the geographic area where you want to live).

Assessing Occupational Preferences and Your Skills

Regardless of what stage of career planning you are in, a good way to help you identify your occupational preferences, skills and abilities, and aptitude is taking some **personal assessments.** Career counselors, placement coordinators, and educational advisers have access to a variety of assessments to help you make decisions. Assessments are like insurance policies—they help ensure you're headed in whatever direction is right for you and you're adequately prepared to tackle the next step in your career plan.

It's important to plan ahead, take one step at a time, and avoid rushing into a situation for which you aren't prepared. Make sure you have the knowledge and skills you need to be a well-qualified match for your next job. You're acquiring the theoretical knowledge, technical hands-on skills, and fundamental experience you'll need for your first, entry-level job now. It's also a good idea to make sure your **basic skills** are up to speed to support continued growth, both professionally and personally. Once again, this is where personal assessments can help. Work with an adult basic education instructor to assess your basic skills (i.e., reading, writing, English, public speaking, and math) and help you overcome any deficiencies. Expect to revisit the need to strengthen basic skills at each stage of your career. If you wish to advance into a leadership role, writing and verbal communication skills will be paramount. And it's not unusual for health care workers to need a math refresher when moving into a new job that requires a different type of math application. Reading and English comprehension are other basic skills that may benefit from enhancement now and then.

How well developed are your computer skills? To function in today's world and to advance in your career, computer skills are no longer optional—they're a necessity. Most health care facilities now rely on computers to process and transmit medical and financial information and to communicate with insurance companies, suppliers, vendors, and other business partners. Health care networks use sophisticated software for patient charting and to enter patient requisitions, schedule procedures, and document test results. Health care companies are increasingly becoming "paperless" using technology to store and transfer vital information. Hospitals publish web sites to provide information for consumers and to link employees with personal information such as timecard records, payroll data, and employee benefits. Hospitals use computers to enroll employees in educational offerings, document compliance with mandatory learning requirements, and produce transcripts of course completions. Annual performance evaluations may require entering performance ratings into on-line forms. Every year, more and more functions become computerized. The young students of today may have mastered the use of computers by the time they start **postsecondary** education, but many adult students and workers have yet to learn these skills. If you don't have basic computer skills yourself, it's time to learn. Once you've mastered the basics, you'll be off and running, eager to learn more. Computer literacy is not only a "basic skill" in today's world, it's a great way to increase efficiency, build confidence and self-esteem, connect with other people throughout the world, and acquire infinite sources of information.

Another way to assess your knowledge and skills is to ask for feedback from people who are familiar with you and your work. How you view yourself and the quality of your work might be different from other people's impressions of you. Learn all you can about the impression you make on others and look for ways to improve. Ask your program director, instructors, and other people who've been involved in your education for feedback on your performance. What do they view as your strengths and your areas for improvement? How do they describe your interpersonal, organizational, communication, and problem-solving skills? What advice might they offer to help you to prepare for employment? Although you may hear some negative comments, view this feedback as **constructive criticism,** geared to make you an even better professional. This will give you some valuable experience for the more in-depth and formal performance evaluations you can expect once you are on the job. When it comes time to apply for a job, a positive recommendation from the people at your school could be extremely important.

Exploring Employment Opportunities

Where are the best employment opportunities that match your interests and abilities? Investigate hospitals but don't forget to also look into outpatient facilities; home care agencies; community health clinics; rehabilitation facilities; physician practices; mental health centers; public health organizations; and satellite imaging, laboratory, and surgery centers. You might be surprised at the variety of places that employ people with your education and skills. Get in the habit of reading the classified advertisements in local newspapers and track job opportunities from week to week. Surf the Internet and check out professional association and employer web sites. Peruse occupational reference materials. Talk with other health care workers to get their opinions on the best places to work. Ask a school librarian or placement specialist to help you track down current employment trends. Meet with human resources personnel to learn all you can about job openings, salary ranges, employment benefits, and opportunities for career development. Identify which employers provide support for career advancement such as scholarships, tuition reimbursement, on-site continuing education, advanced training programs, and flexible work schedules to accommodate employees who return to school. If an employer has already helped you with a scholarship, part-time job, or some other means of support while you've been in school, remember the discussion earlier in this book about loyalty. If the employer "took a chance" on you and invested in your education, then you have an obligation to "re-pay" that investment. Professionals fulfill their commitments.

Networking with a variety of people can help you strengthen your interpersonal skills and learn about job opportunities and the best places to work. Join a professional association, become a volunteer, or participate in community activities to hone your communication skills, meet new people, and widen your scope of collegial relationships and friendships.

This is no time to shirk on your homework. Spend some extra time assessing your strengths, improving your skills, making contacts with other people who can help you, and investigating the best employment opportunities. Making good decisions early in your career increases your potential for a lifetime filled with satisfying and rewarding work.

Setting Goals

Once you've explored your occupational interests, taken advantage of assessments, enhanced your skills, and identified the best employment opportunities, it's time to set goals for the next phase of your career. As mentioned in Chapter One, goals are well-defined stepping-stones that help you progress from where you are now to where you eventually want to be. Short-term goals are those attained in a relatively brief period of time—up to about two years—whereas long-term goals take much longer. Long-term goals often involve meeting some short-term goals along the way. For example, if you're in nursing school now and your long-term goal is to become a nurse practitioner, your short-term goals might include taking prerequisite courses and saving more money for tuition and books. If you're in a surgical technology program and aspire to eventually become a surgical nurse, you might find an evening shift job so you can attend nursing classes and clinical rotations during the day. If you're in a medical assisting program and aspire to become an office manager, you might seek a job with opportunities to gain leadership skills and supervisory experience. If you're in a hospital-based radiography program and eventually want to earn a bachelor's degree in diagnostic imaging, you might enroll in a college and start taking liberal arts and sciences courses.

It's important to envision your future and "stretch" to your potential, but it's also important to set realistic, attainable goals that are right for you. **Role models** and **mentors** can help. Role models are people who already have the kind of abilities, education, job, and professional reputation that you aspire to achieve yourself. Obviously, you can learn a lot from a role model because that person has already traveled down the road you are just starting out on. Get to know your role model, observe what makes him or her successful, and decide if the approach your role model took would also work for you. Working with a mentor can be a big help, too. Unlike role models, mentors have not necessarily achieved the same goals you hope to achieve. But mentors can provide you with insight, advice, and encouragement to help you each step of the way. While on the subject of role models and mentors, it's important for you to serve as a role model and mentor for other people, too. Remember, we're all on this road together. Just as others are helping you reach your goals, you can help other people reach theirs.

Balancing Priorities and Career Advancement

As you set goals and proceed with your career plan, it's important to adjust your priorities and your work schedule to balance your personal and professional lives. Avoid overloading yourself. It's better to take more time and do well than to rush things and do poorly. Taking one step at a time is good advice. Finding time to do the things you enjoy in life is important, especially spending time with your family. It's not unusual to hear people wonder whether the time they're spending on work and career advancement is negatively effecting their families. They know they're setting good examples for their children by demonstrating the value of self-discipline and hard work, yet balancing priorities and the demands of a dynamic career can be a challenge for most any health care professional. Achieving your goals and reaping the benefits of a successful health career may require some adjustments.

Don't be surprised if your goals change over time and don't become discouraged if attaining a goal takes longer than you had anticipated. Adjustments and delays are part of the process as you learn more about yourself, what you want out of your career, and what's going to work best for you and your family. The important thing is that you have a career plan with realistic goals and you're on the road to where you eventually want to be.

Expecting the Unexpected

Chapter Four discussed the importance of adapting to change and letting change open new doors for you. Even if you've established some goals and are well on your way to achieving them, keep your eyes open for new opportunities when you least expect them. Today's health care system is in the midst of rapid change. Jobs are being redesigned, departments are being reorganized, and some types of health care services are moving from the hospital setting to outpatient facilities. Increasing numbers of workers are being trained, cross-trained, and retrained for new responsibilities. Even if your current goals don't call for additional training, your employer might require gaining new skills as part of a work redesign or organizational restructuring initiative. If this type of opportunity comes your way, seize it and make it work to your advantage. Health care professionals must be lifelong learners, always acquiring new knowledge, skills, and responsibilities to benefit themselves and the patients they serve.

Expect to take some risks along the way. Risk taking *does not* mean being foolish or haphazard in how you make decisions. But it *does* mean taking some well-thought-out, calculated steps that force you to stretch a little bit. After all, if you don't try, you'll never know if you could have been successful. If your goals are realistic, if you take things one step at a time, and if you apply yourself and do your best, then you stand a good chance of eventually arriving at where you want to be.

If the going gets rough, don't give up. Talk with your role model, mentor, family members, or friends for encouragement and support. You'll probably hear that just about everyone else thought about giving up at one time or another. If your goals are worth achieving, they're worth fighting for. Hang in there.

Résumés

Once you've established your goals and are ready to seek a new job, preparing a résumé will likely be part of the process. Even if you lack substantial postsecondary education and work experience, it's still a good idea to have a résumé. Résumés give employers a snapshot of your background and the qualifications you're presenting for consideration. Résumés also provide visible evidence of your written communication skills. If you've never developed a résumé, use the Student CD-ROM that comes with this text for help. You can also locate books in your school library or local bookstore to give you some guidance and examples. Or ask someone who writes or reviews résumés to assist you. (Refer to the Appendix for a sample résumé.)

Your résumé should be typed, professional in appearance, concise, and able to be electronically scanned, sent as an email attachment, or photocopied with good quality. Use white paper and avoid fancy, colored paper with borders or graphic designs. Organize the information and make sure your grammar and spelling are correct. Emphasize your educational background and your skills and abilities that match the qualifications for the job. If you're a young person with little or no occupational experience and limited postsecondary education, it's OK to list some of your high school accomplishments and extracurricular activities such as academic awards, sports, orchestra or choir, science fair entries, perfect attendance awards, or participation in school organizations. If you served in a leadership role in a school organization, be sure to include that. If it's an accomplishment you are proud of, go ahead and list it. Also list your computer skills, seminars or training sessions you've attended, certificates you've earned, and any distinctions or awards you've received. Develop a well-written cover letter to accompany your résumé. (Refer to the Appendix for a sample résumé cover letter.)

Submitting supportive documents with your résumé (e.g., copies of certificates, grade transcripts, or recommendation letters from an instructor or your family physician) is usually permissible but don't get carried away. Select one or two of the best to submit with your résumé and save the others for your interview in case you get a chance to present them in person. And don't be surprised if employers require you to submit your résumé and an employment application on-line. Increasing numbers of employers are using "paperless" application and employment procedures.

Job Application Forms

As with the résumé, the job application form conveys a lot of information about you and is an important part of the employment process. If employers receive a surplus of applications for a particular job opening, the application form is typically the first item they use to narrow down the applicant pool and "screen out" applicants. Employers screen applications to evaluate how well your qualifications match those of the job. They determine how well you can read and follow directions and they assess your written communication skills (including spelling and grammar) and your neatness. (Refer to the Appendix for a sample job application form.)

If required to submit your application on-line, allow time to become familiar with the company's computer software and don't hesitate to ask for help if you need it. If the company requests a paper application form, make sure you fill it out yourself instead of asking someone to do it for you. It's best to type the information. If you don't type, make sure your writing is legible and neat. Read and follow the directions for filling out the application form. Make sure all words are spelled correctly and list accurate dates for your education and work experience. Review the form to make sure you haven't left anything out. If the application calls for a brief statement about why you're applying for the job, take some time to think about your answer before writing it. You'd be surprised how much weight your answer might carry in the selection process.

Use your best written communication skills. Convince the reviewers that you're familiar with the job and the company. Let them know you believe that they offer a good match for you and your abilities and interests. If space permits, describe briefly how hiring you would benefit the employer. Your job application and accompanying résumé make that all-important first impression. Spend a sufficient amount of time making sure it's the impression you want conveyed. These two documents will likely determine whether you get invited in for an interview or not.

Most people have a tendency to "undersell" themselves so it's important to present your best attributes. But stand on your own merits. Never exaggerate or falsify any of the information. Misrepresentation is dishonest and constitutes fraud. It's unprofessional, unethical, and likely to result in your dismissal should your lies ever be discovered. If you've had a misdemeanor or felony conviction, you must disclose it on a job application. Most employers do criminal history background checks as part of the employment process. A prior conviction may or may not eliminate you from consideration, depending on the type of offense, how long ago it occurred, and so forth. But if you fail to disclose the conviction and your employer discovers it later on, it could be grounds for immediate dismissal.

Employers are now searching the Internet to gather additional information on job applicants. They may "Google" your name, view your web site, read your blog, and review other information that you or someone else has published about you. This is public information so be careful about what you publish.

Most employers require references. Choose your references carefully. One reference should be qualified to attest to your knowledge, abilities, and potential for learning, such as a program director, instructor, or supervisor. You may need to provide written permission before your program faculty or supervisors can disclose information about your performance. Another reference should be qualified to comment on your character, work ethic, and reliability. Be sure to contact these individuals first and ask for permission to list them as references. Let them know what job you're applying for and when they might expect to be contacted by the employer. Select people who are not only familiar with your skills and the quality of your work, but who also have positive, insightful, and complimentary things to say about you. The more credible the reference, the better. Never use relatives as references. Mentors and role models can be helpful, either as references themselves or as advisors in résumé writing and navigating the employment process.

As mentioned previously, one of the most frequent reasons for terminating employees is poor attendance, so employers are especially interested in the attendance record of job applicants. Hiring managers are typically impressed by job applicants who have demonstrated their time management skills and their ability to balance school, a job, and a personal life with good results. When an employer contacts your references for feedback about your performance and reliability, expect your attendance to be one of the topics discussed.

If you know someone who works for the company to which you are applying, and if that person is familiar with you and the quality of your work, consider listing him or her as a reference. But avoid "name dropping," "pulling strings," or "using connections" to try to enhance your chances of a job offer. Such attempts could have a negative effect on hiring managers and back-fire on you. Take the professional approach—stand on your own merits and get hired for the right reasons.

Pre-Employment Assessments

Don't be surprised if you're asked to take some written or computerized assessments as part of the employment process. Employers need to know if you're qualified for the job and match the characteristics of the type of employees they prefer to hire. Some require on-line assessments while others schedule half-day or full-day assessments to evaluate your: (1) basic skills such as reading, writing, English, and math; (2) work ethic, character, personal values, personality traits, and customer service skills; and (3) specific job-related skills such as a typing, computer literacy, applied math, and so forth.

Pre-employment assessments are difficult to prepare for because they measure the accumulation of the knowledge, skills, and personal characteristics that you've developed over an extended period of time. Try not to be intimidated by these kinds of assessments. Get plenty of sleep the night before to be well rested, eat a good breakfast, and concentrate on doing your best. Afterward, if possible, ask for some feedback on how well you performed so you'll be aware of your strong and weak points. If scores indicate some weaknesses, work on strengthening these areas as you apply for other jobs. If you don't get an interview the first time you apply, you can enhance your qualifications and reapply later.

Most of today's health care jobs require either a high school diploma or a General Equivalency Diploma (GED) plus successful completion of postsecondary education or training. There are still a limited number of jobs for people without a high school diploma or a GED, but until you earn one or the other, you are locked in an entry-level job with little or no opportunities for advancement. Depending on the job for which you are applying, employers will require verification of your educational background. You may need to submit an **official transcript** or copies of diplomas, certificates of completion, or college degrees. You may also be instructed to submit verification of professional certifications, licenses, registrations, or other credentials required for the job.

Preparing for an Interview

Once you've submitted your job application form, résumé, and supportive documentation and survived the first screening, you're ready to prepare for your personal interview. Making a good impression during an interview pulls together just about everything discussed in this book. The objective is to present yourself as a qualified, motivated, caring professional who is well prepared for the job. Interviewers will be looking for information about your academic achievements, occupational experience, interpersonal skills, and personal qualities to help decide if you are a good fit for the company and the position. Don't just show up for an interview. Do your homework first.

Learn as much as you can about the job and the employer ahead of time so you can talk intelligently about the opportunity for which you are applying. For example, if you're applying for a job in an outpatient clinic, find out what kinds of patients are seen there, what services are provided on site, what kinds of workers are employed there, what hours the clinic is open, and so on. If you appear for an interview and aren't familiar with basic information about the company, interviewers will wonder if you're really serious about being hired or not. If you take the time to investigate the company first, interviewers are more likely to be impressed with your interest and may give you some extra consideration.

Even if you've already answered the question about why you're applying for the job on the application form, you'll probably be asked this question again during the interview. Knowing as much as you can about the job for which you are applying will help convince interviewers that you've given this question a lot of thought and that you're sure you're a good match for the opening. Someone may ask exactly *what* you did to investigate the job or the company to make sure they are what you're looking for. If you've done your homework, you'll have several examples to share with interviewers.

Interviewers use traditional and behavioral questioning techniques. With traditional questioning, they're asking how you *would* behave given certain circumstances. With behavioral questioning, they're asking how you *did* behave, believing that past performance is the best predictor of future performance. Here are some examples to illustrate the difference.

> Traditional: "What are your strengths and weaknesses?"
>
> Behavioral: "Describe a weakness that you experienced in your past and tell me what you did to overcome it."
>
> Traditional: "How do you handle pressure and stress?"
>
> Behavioral: "Describe a stressful situation and how you handled it."

Behavioral interview questions are more probing and call for specific answers. Instead of asking, "What are your goals for the next five years?" the question might be, "What were your goals when you started school and how successful were you in accomplishing them?" Once you've answered a behavioral question, expect more detailed followup questions. "What did you do or say that led to that outcome?" "Why did you try that approach?" Prepare for both types of questions since you won't know until you get there what approach the interviewer will use. It could be a combination of both. Refresh your memory about special challenges you have faced, projects you have worked on, and goals you have achieved. Have some personal stories in mind in case you're asked for examples. Knowing as much as you can about the job description and the skills that your interviewer is seeking will help you anticipate the types of questions that might be asked.

Practice at home with someone firing questions at you in a mock interview setting. Be prepared to answer questions such as the following:

Why are you interested in this job?

Have you ever had a job that didn't turn out to be what you expected? What did you do about it?

What specifically have you done to investigate this job?

How can you be sure if this job is right for you?

Have you ever been fired from a job? If so, why were you fired and how did you react?

Have you experienced conflict with a former supervisor? If so, how did you resolve it?

What do you think it would take to be successful in this job?

What have you done to prepare yourself for this job?

Did you have to learn something new in your previous job? If so, how did you do that?

What strengths would you bring to this job and this company?

How did you support the reputation of the company you used to work for?

What appeals to you about working for this company?

Why should we select you over other applicants?

Have you ever applied for a job and didn't get it? If so, what did you do?

What will you do if you're not selected for this job?

The more questions you can anticipate in advance, the better prepared you will be. Expect some "what if?" questions such as, "What would you do if you had to be late for work one morning?" or "What would you do if you observed a coworker stealing from the company?"

The night before your interview, read this section of this chapter again so everything is fresh in your mind and you're ready to go. Get plenty of sleep and eat a good breakfast or lunch before your appointment. Make sure you know exactly where to go, how to get there, and where to park. Plan to arrive at least 20 minutes early. If something unforeseen occurs and you are unable to be there at the appointed time, call and let the appropriate person know. Allow plenty of time for the interview itself. Other applicants may be scheduled for interviews during the same time period as you, so interviewers could be running late and you might be kept waiting. It should go without saying but must be mentioned—don't bring your children with you to an interview! Having children present is disruptive and an indication that you lack reliable childcare.

Participating in an Interview

Once you've prepared for the interview and appeared at the right time and place, it's important to make a positive, professional impression. Start by looking your very best. If you're wearing a uniform as part of your externship or clinical rotations and your interview takes place just before, after, or during your assigned hours, either take a change of clothing to wear for the interview or make absolutely certain your uniform is impeccably clean and pressed and your hair is well groomed. Avoid clothes, hairstyles, or other visible signs that might distract interviewers or elicit an undesirable reaction. Examples include miniskirts, low-cut blouses, saggy pants, flip flop shoes, hair that glows in the dark, tattoos, and facial and/or tongue piercings. You want to make a lasting impression on interviewers based on your qualifications, not your outlandish appearance. Good grooming is essential, including clean hair, clean fingernails, and polished shoes. Make sure your breath is fresh and use deodorant. Don't show up with blood shot eyes or smelling of alcohol or cigarette smoke. Think twice about long, brightly colored fingernails; they aren't acceptable in many types of health care jobs. Keep jewelry and accessories to a minimum and avoid fragrances. Men may want to rethink wearing earrings. Review Chapter Four to refresh your memory on details regarding professional appearance.

Be sure to bring copies of your résumé, a list of references with their contact information, and a notepad and pen. On the notepad, list a few of your personal accomplishments and some notes about the stories you've recalled so you'll have them fresh in your mind in case you are asked. Jot down an example of how you've handled stress in the past and a situation where you had to learn something new, just in case you're asked for examples. Have at least two questions prepared that you want to ask the interviewer when the opportunity arises. Two good questions might be, "What's the potential for growth and advancement within your company?" and "What characteristics are you looking for in the ideal candidate for this job?" If you dropped out of school or left previous jobs, be prepared to explain why.

In Chapter One you read about the value of keeping a binder to use during your annual performance evaluation. Suggested items include "thank you's" from coworkers, patients, or physicians; awards or citations that you have received; transcripts of continuing education, classes and courses you've completed; copies of professional certifications you've earned; and other evidence of your performance and professional growth. If you have items such as these from school, a previous job, volunteer experiences, or activities in the community, consider bringing copies of the most relevant items with you to your interview.

SMILE! Smiling is one of the easiest ways to make a good first impression. Offer a firm handshake and try to remember the names of the people who are introduced to you. Apply your best interpersonal communication skills and personality traits. Remember the importance of customer service? All health care employers seek people with pleasant personalities who can relate well to other people. Practice your best people skills. It's OK to be nervous—in fact interviewers might wonder what's wrong with you if you aren't nervous. But try to maintain your composure and self-confidence.

Let interviewers know what skills and abilities you would bring to the job. Convince them that you can make a positive contribution to their organization and serve as an effective member of their team. Remember why you chose a career in health care? Let your enthusiasm and commitment to helping people show. Be sincere. Don't just fabricate statements that you think interviewers want to hear. If you've done an adequate job of preparing for your interview, you've identified some good examples of your personal and professional traits to share with interviewers. Be yourself. Don't pretend to be someone you *think* would be more appealing to the interviewers. You want the job to be right for you and you want yourself to be right for the job. Trust the interviewers to recognize a good match when they see one.

Be honest! Employers check references, criminal histories, and licensing and educational records. If you're asked why you left school or terminated employment, tell the truth. Employers are especially interested in attendance and may ask you about your attendance records in school and on the job. They may ask if you have reliable transportation.

Sit up straight, don't chew gum or bite your fingernails, and try to relax! Pay attention to your body language and the non-verbal messages you are sending. Convey a positive attitude. This is not a time to express anger or frustration from a former job or supervisor. Don't carry "baggage" from your past into what could become a new situation and fresh start. Display self-confidence and a genuine interest in what's being discussed.

Even if you decide early in the interview that you aren't interested in the job, continue to "put your best foot forward." A few years from now you may want to apply there again. The person who interviews you at one company may know the people who do the hiring at other companies. Never pass up an opportunity to make a good impression.

Some interview sessions are quite formal while others are more conversational and informal. If you're invited to lunch or dinner, don't let your guard down because it feels like a social setting. You are still being "sized-up" as a potential employee. Don't be surprised if you're interviewed by more than one person, perhaps at the same time. Having one person fire questions at you can be intimidating enough without having two or three people doing the same thing during the same session. Sometimes employers have no choice but to have multiple people interview an applicant at the same time. Occasionally, it's done intentionally to see how well an applicant performs under pressure.

Concentrate on each question and think before you answer. Don't just blurt out the first thought that pops into your head. But don't ponder the question for too long either. Interviewers want to know if you can think and analyze situations quickly. Having some answers already formulated in your mind will help. Let your interviewer know that you are always eager to learn new things. As was mentioned previously, health care changes rapidly. Companies seek employees who adapt well to change, learn new things quickly, and readily accept cross-training and additional new job duties. Sometimes interviewers will ask questions just to see how you perform under stress. Expect this to happen and don't let these kinds of questions shake your confidence.

To prevent discrimination in the selection process, there are several questions that interviewers are not supposed to ask. These relate to personal characteristics such as your age, ethnicity, physical condition, religion, lifestyle preferences (heterosexual, homosexual, bisexual), marital status, and plans for either starting or expanding your family (i.e., pregnancies). Unfortunately, some interviewers do ask inappropriate questions, so it's important to anticipate these questions and have a response in mind. If, for example, an interviewer asks a female applicant, "When do you plan to start a family?" she might reply, "Having a family is important to me but so is a successful career. I know that balancing your professional and personal lives is a challenge. But I worked two part-time jobs and helped take care of my elderly grandmother while I was completing my education so I know I can manage my time."

The interviewing process is not a one-way street—it's OK for you to ask questions, too. In fact, many interviewers expect applicants to ask questions. When your questions are answered, jot down the responses along with any other information you don't want to forget. Interviewers will notice that you are organized, pay attention to details, and record important information. Avoid asking questions that are already answered in printed materials or web sites that were available to you in advance. If you ask a question that's already been answered in some other obvious place, interviewers may wonder if you even read the material. As mentioned earlier, two good questions might be, "What's the potential for growth and advancement within your company?" and "What characteristics are you looking for in the ideal candidate for this job?" The first question lets the interviewer know that you're ambitious and seeking a company that you can grow with. The second question gives you valuable information and the opportunity to explain how your qualifications match what the interviewer is seeking.

Not everyone agrees on whether or not to ask questions about pay and benefits during the first interview. Although pay and benefits are important, it's best to focus on the primary responsibilities of the job and the qualifications being sought by the employer. If you know there's going to be a second, follow-up interview, wait for that appointment to ask about pay and benefits. Or, let the interviewer take the lead in bringing up the discussion during your first interview. Give some thought ahead of time to what your pay and benefit requirements would be in case you are asked those questions during your first interview. Saying, "I don't know" or "I haven't really thought about it" indicates you haven't done your homework. Remember the advice given earlier in this chapter. Before your interview, investigate customary pay ranges for the job you are seeking by using occupational reference materials or talking with a placement advisor at school or a human resources consultant or manager where you would be working. How much pay do you need? It's OK to say, "It's negotiable" but have an acceptable range in mind in case you get pinned down or a job offer is extended. If you've done your homework, you've already identified what's most important in selecting the best offer. Instead of focusing on starting pay and benefits, new graduates should probably be more concerned about the job itself, support for continuing education, and opportunities to gain new skills and valuable work experience.

Whether or not you still want the job, you should follow-up the interview with a letter thanking the employer for the opportunity to interview. This demonstrates courtesy and good manners and it also puts your name and communication skills in front of the decision-makers one more time. Delivering a hand-written thank you letter or sending a thank-you email message within 24 hours after your interview will make a good impression since the majority of job applicants fail to follow-up. Your "thank you" correspondence also provides an opportunity to restate how excited you are about joining the company and to follow-up on something discussed or forgotten during the interview. (Refer to the Appendix for a sample interview follow-up letter.)

If you do want the job, also telephone the interviewer and ask if there is anything else you can do to verify your qualifications or answer any remaining questions. Try to wait patiently. It can take several weeks before employment decisions are finalized and offers are made. Avoid calling the interviewer frequently to ask if a decision has been made yet. You don't want to become an annoyance or appear desperate. Most companies will notify all candidates when a position has been filled.

If selected for the job, you can expect to undergo a drug screen as part of your pre-employment physical examination. Employers can ill afford to hire people with substance abuse problems. This is one example of a "first impression" where you won't be given a second chance.

Pull together everything you've learned about professionalism and apply it to the résumé writing, application, and interviewing process. Expect some competition with other job applicants. The supply and demand for workers varies over time, often occurring in cycles. When employers face shortages of qualified workers, it's easier for qualified candidates to secure jobs and they may have several job offers from which to choose. But when there's a surplus of qualified job candidates for the number of positions available, competition can be fierce.

If you get the job you desire, you'll be on the road to achieving another goal. If you don't get selected, you'll know you did your best and you will have learned something in the process. If you feel you are truly qualified, don't give up. Employers value perseverance. Ask for feedback on how to enhance your qualifications. Then follow the advice and reapply. It's not unusual for applicants to be turned down the first time and then hired later on. If you reapply and are turned down a second time, work with an adviser or mentor to revisit your goals and identify ways to increase your qualifications. If you're seeking employment in a large or specialized facility or in a city or town where the competition for jobs is formidable, consider applying for a job in a smaller facility or in another city or town first and then making a move later on. Gaining work experience with a good reference someplace else may be the key to securing the job you really want.

Never underestimate the importance of obtaining a professional credential, even when not required for employment. Securing a license, certification, or registration verifies that you have met the education and competency standards set forth by a professional organization or governmental agency. Employers can rest assured that you have the knowledge and skills necessary to perform the duties of your job in a safe and quality-oriented manner.

Once you've graduated and landed your job, don't think you're done with education. Nothing could be farther from the truth! Working in health care requires life-long learning. Medicine and health care constantly advance, and your knowledge and skills must advance to keep up with the pace. As mentioned in Chapter One, health care professionals are expected to keep up with current trends and issues both on the local and national levels. People will expect you to know what's going on in your industry and be able to talk intelligently about it. Read articles in newspapers and magazines, watch the news on television, monitor newsworthy web sites, and be on the lookout for special programs and reports.

More than likely, your employer will expect you to undergo more training at work when new equipment, supplies, and computer systems are implemented or when your job duties expand or change. As you work towards advancement, you'll need to acquire additional knowledge and skills to perform your new responsibilities. You may wish to return to school and work towards advanced degrees or earn additional professional certifications. Your employer may send you to some outside conferences or training sessions to learn something new with the expectation that you will summarize your learning and pass the information on to your coworkers when you return.

Expect to attend in-service sessions, participate in local and national continuing education seminars, and read professional journals throughout your health career. Many health care professions now mandate continuing education as a requirement for maintaining professional certifications, registrations, or licenses. The specific requirements for mandatory continuing education vary among the different professions so it's important to become familiar with the requirements for your profession. Some professions even require periodic re-testing to make sure that people are maintaining their competencies. One of the best ways to maintain your knowledge and skills over the years is to become active in your professional associations. Not only will you have access to upcoming continuing education offerings, you'll also have opportunities to network with other professionals and gain experience working on committees and serving in elected leadership roles. Active membership in professional associations also gives you a voice and the chance to influence where your profession is headed in the future. How much do you know about the history of your profession and its future outlook? Over the years you will invest a great deal of time, effort, and personal resources in your professional endeavors. The future of your profession, and what it can offer you years from now, is in the hands of people just like you.

Don't think that you can graduate from school, land a good job, and then rest on your laurels. Health care professionals with dynamic careers always have more things to learn and more goals to achieve. The final "In Summary" section of this text provides some inspiration for your journey.

L E A R N I N G   A C T I V I T I E S

Using information from Chapter Six:

❑ Respond to the What If? Scenarios below

❑ Answer the Review Questions below

❑ Watch the video for Chapter Six on the accompanying Student CD-ROM and complete the CD-ROM Assignments

What If? Scenarios

Think about what you would do in the following situations and record your answers.

1. You've just graduated from school, moved to a new town, and need to find a good job. But you don't know anyone in town and you aren't familiar with area health care employers.

2. A new job just opened up but it requires some extra math skills. You're interested in applying but don't know if your math is strong enough to meet the qualifications.

3. You're meeting with your supervisor for your annual performance review and you might get some negative feedback.

4. You're planning to apply for a new job but your résumé is four years old. The new job is somewhat different from the one you have now but some of your skills might be transferable.

5. You have a job interview at 8 a.m. Saturday morning. Your friends are having a party Friday night that starts at 9 p.m. and they want you to join them.

6. The job for which you would like to apply requires five years of previous work experience. You have three years of work experience in a large hospital that, to you, seems comparable to five years in a smaller hospital. A small change on your résumé would make you appear eligible to apply even though it wouldn't be totally accurate.

7. Last semester, your grade-point average dropped to a 2.0 (on a 4.0 scale) because you missed several classes while taking care of an injured family member. The company where you've applied for a job wants a copy of your transcript to verify your graduation. Because the company did not require an official transcript, it would be easy to change the 2.0 GPA to a 3.0. After all, your grades would have been better if not for missing several classes due to a family emergency.

8. After deciding to apply for a new job in an outpatient clinic, you find out your mother knows the clinic's human resource manager. Just a few months ago, your mother helped him refinance his home mortgage and your mother has offered to make a phone call to the human resources manager on your behalf.

9. The only interview appointment that's open is at 4 p.m. on Wednesday. You're scheduled to work at your current job up until 3:30 p.m. that day. Your supervisor has told you and your coworkers to wear old clothes that day because you'll be moving supplies and setting up a new inventory room.

10. You've applied for the same job twice and have yet to be selected.

Review Questions

Using information from Chapter Six, answer each of the following.

1. Explain the difference between a stagnant career and a dynamic career.

2. List five questions to ask yourself in career planning and identify three helpful resources.

3. Describe personal assessments and what you can learn from them.

4. List four ways to explore employment opportunities where you live.

5. Define *goals, short-term goals, long-term goals,* and *realistic goals* and explain why goals are important.

6. Describe role models and mentors and explain their value.

7. Identify the importance of computer skills in career advancement.

8. Explain the importance of job application forms and identify four factors in completing them appropriately.

9. Describe the role of pre-employment assessments.

10. List five important factors in participating in a job interview.

11. Describe why continuing education is important for health care workers and list two ways to obtain continuing education.

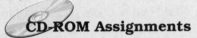 **CD-ROM Assignments**

Select Chapter Six on the accompanying Student CD-ROM and complete the assignments.

In Summary

Expect to encounter many bumps on the road to professional success. Some you will navigate quite handily while others require more maneuvering. At times you will soar, and now and then you will stumble and, perhaps, even fall. After all, we are all just less-than-perfect human beings trying to do our very best. Learn from your successes and your failures. Challenge yourself to always improve. Put your patients first and treat everyone with respect and compassion. Face your future with courage and conviction, pause to appreciate the small things in life, and enjoy each and every step of your journey. Best wishes for a stellar health career!

"It is not the critic who counts, not the man who points out how the strong man stumbled, or where the doer of deeds could have done better. The credit belongs to the man who is actually in the arena, whose face is marred by dust and sweat and blood, who strives valiantly, who errs and comes short again and again, who knows the great enthusiasms, the great devotions, and spends himself in a worthy cause, who at best knows achievement and who at the worst if he fails at least fails while daring greatly so that his place shall never be with those cold and timid souls who know neither victory nor defeat."

Theodore Roosevelt, 26th U.S. President, 1858–1919

Glossary of Terms

accountable   accepts responsibility and the consequences of one's actions 7

adaptive skills   the ability to adjust to change 88

basic skills   fundamental aptitudes in reading, language, and math 122

body language   nonverbal messages communicated by posture, hand gestures, facial expressions, etc. 52

caregivers   health care workers who provide direct, hands-on patient care 3

certification   a credential from a state agency or a professional association awarding permission to use a special professional title; must meet pre-established competency standards 16

character   a person's moral behavior and qualities 26

cliques   small, exclusive circles of people 42

colleagues   fellow workers in the same profession 43

competence   possessing necessary knowledge and skills 9

confidentiality   maintaining the privacy of certain matters 5

conflict of interest   an inappropriate relationship between personal interests and official responsibilities 14

conflict resolution   overcoming disagreements between two or more people 52

conscience   moral judgment that prohibits or opposes the violation of a previously recognized ethical principle 28

consensus   decision that all members agree to support 46

constructive criticism   viewing one's weaknesses in a way that leads to positive improvement 123

contingency plans   backup plans in case the original plans don't work 6

corporate compliance   acting in accordance with laws and with a company's rules, policies, and procedures 14

corporate mission   special duties, functions, or purposes of a company 17

corporate values   beliefs held in high esteem by a company 17

corrective action   steps taken to overcome a job performance problem 6

critical thinking   using careful analysis and objective judgment 86

diligent   careful in one's work 9

discretion   being careful about what one says and does 18

dismissal   involuntary termination from a job 6

diversity   differences, dissimilarities, variations 47

dress code   standards for attire and appearance 74

dynamic   in motion, energetic and vigorous 120

empathetic   relating to another person's emotions and situation 60

ethics   standards of conduct and moral judgment 28

etiquette   acceptable standards of behavior 107

fraud   intentional deceit through false information or misrepresentation 31

front-line workers   employees who have the most frequent contact with a company's customers 17

goals   objects or ends that one strives to attain, aims 11

grammar   system of word structures and arrangements 73

group norms   expectations or guidelines for group behavior 46

heterogeneous   different, composed of different elements 44

hierarchy   a group of people or units arranged by rank 5

HIPAA   Health Insurance Portability and Accountability Act of 1996; national standards to protect the privacy of a patient's personal health information 14

homogeneous   the same, composed of similar elements 44

hostile workplace   an uncomfortable or unsafe work environment 14

impaired   a reduced ability to function properly 5

inclusive   a tendency to include everyone 42

insubordination   refusal to complete an assigned task 7

integrity   of sound moral principle 27

interdepartmental teams   groups of people from different departments 44

interdependence   the need to rely on one another 41

interdisciplinary teams   groups of people from different disciplines 44

interpersonal relationships   connections between or among people 41

intradepartmental teams   groups of people from within the same department 44

intradisciplinary teams   groups of people from within the same discipline 44

job shadowing   observing workers to see what their jobs are like 121

journal   a private, written record of a person's thoughts and experiences 105

judgment   comparison of options to decide which is best 28

license   a credential from a state agency awarding legal permission to practice; must meet pre-established qualifications 15

loyal   faithful to people that one is under obligation to defend or support 42

manners   standards of behavior based on thoughtfulness and consideration of other people 51

mentors   wise, loyal advisers 125

morals   capability of differentiating between right and wrong 27

multiskilled   cross-trained to perform more than one function, often in more than one discipline 46

networking   interacting with a variety of people in different settings 124

objective   what is real or actual; not affected by feelings 10

observations   on-site learning experiences for students to view a "real-life" setting and take note of what occurs there 104

occupational preferences   the types of work and work settings that an individual prefers 121

office politics   clique-like relationships among groups of coworkers that involve scheming and plotting 107

official transcript   grade report that is printed, sealed, and mailed directly to the recipient to prevent tampering by the applicant 129

organizational chart   illustration showing the components of a company and how they fit together 5

optimists   people who look on the bright side of things 8

peers   people at the same rank 11

performance evaluation   measurement of success in executing job duties 10

penmanship   handwriting 112

personal assessments   questionnaires and tests that identify interests and evaluate abilities 122

personal financial management   the ability to make sound decisions about personal finances 81

personal image   the total impression created by a person 73

personal management skills   the ability to manage time, finances, stress, and change 79

personal skills   the ability to manage aspects of your life outside of work 73

personal values   things of great worth and importance 26

perspective   the manner in which a person views something 8

pessimists   people who look on the dark side of things 8

postsecondary   after high school 123

potential   an ability that can, but has not yet, come into being 120

practicum   a "real-life" learning experience obtained through working on-site in a health care facility while enrolled as a student (other terms: clinicals, externship, internship, hands-on experience, on-site learning, experiential learning) 89

priorities   having precedence in time, order, and importance 28

probationary period   a testing or trial period to meet requirements 11

problem solving   using a systematic process to solve problems 86

profane   improper and contemptible 109

project teams   groups of people who meet for a specified period of time and disband when their project has been completed 44

punctual   arriving for work on time 6

reliable   can be counted upon; trustworthy 7

reputation   a person's character, values, and behavior as viewed by others 27

respect   feeling or showing honor or esteem 29

role models   people that a person aspires to be like 125

samples room   a place where health care facilities keep samples of drugs and medical supplies 107

scope of practice   boundaries that determine what a worker may and may not do as part of his or her job 15

self-esteem   belief in oneself, self-respect 42

self-worth   importance and value in oneself 42

sexual harassment   unwelcome, sexually-oriented advances or comments 14

stagnant   without motion; dull, sluggish 9

stereotype   a fixed or conventional mental pattern 75

stress management   the ability to deal with stress and overcome stressful situations 83

subjective   affected by a state of mind or feelings 10

subordinates   people at a lower rank 10

synergy   people working together in a cooperative action 43

systems perspective   stepping back to view an entire process to see how each component connects with the others 4

time management   the ability to organize and allocate one's time to increase productivity 79

traits   characteristics or qualities related to one's personality 11

transferable skills   skills acquired in one job that are applicable in another job 122

trustworthiness   ability to have confidence in the honesty, integrity, and reliability of another person 27

unethical   a violation of standards of conduct and moral judgment 14

vendors   people who work for companies with which your company does business 3

well groomed   clean and neat 73

whistle blower   a person who exposes the illegal or unethical practices of another person or of a company 17

work ethic   attitudes and behaviors that support good work performance 5

work teams   groups of people who meet on an on-going basis as part of their jobs 44

360-degree feedback   feedback about an employee's job performance that is provided by peers, subordinates, team members, customers, and others who have worked with the employee who is undergoing evaluation 11

Appendix A

HIPAA Overview

Purpose and Scope

The Health Insurance Portability and Accountability Act of 1996 (HIPAA) was enacted to protect the privacy of patients' medical information. Congress instructed the U.S. Department of Health and Human Services (HHS) to issue standards that would provide patients with access to their medical records while giving them more control over how their health information may be used and disclosed. These federal standards took effect on April 14, 2003, and apply uniformly in all states across the country. Privacy regulations limit how identifiable medical information can be used and communicated. While HIPAA provisions encourage electronic transactions, they provide safeguards to protect the security and confidentiality of health information. Pharmacies, physician practices, hospitals, outpatient clinics, health insurance companies, billing companies, and other types of health care providers must comply. Standards apply equally to private, public, and governmental providers. Regulations apply to medical records and other health information conveyed via paper, computers, or orally.

Impact on Patients

Patients must be able to see their medical records, request that corrections be made, and obtain copies as needed. Providers must comply within 30 days and may charge a fee for copying and sending records.

Providers must notify patients of their rights, typically during the patient's first visit. Patients are asked to sign a statement verifying they have been advised of their rights.

Patients may request additional limitations in the use of their medical information beyond what HIPAA mandates. Providers are encouraged to consider such requests but are not required to fulfill them.

Privacy rules allow doctors, nurses, and other health care workers to share information, within limits and as needed, in order to treat patients. Personal health information may not be shared for non-health care purposes, such as marketing, without the patient's written permission.

Individual states may enact state laws to ensure even greater privacy for patients. When a state law requires disclosure of certain types of health information, such as the reporting of an infectious disease, federal privacy standards do not override state law.

Patients may ask their doctors and other health care providers to take additional steps to ensure confidentiality. A patient may ask, for example, that providers avoid conveying personal health information via voicemail messages that could be intercepted by family members or colleagues at work. Providers must make reasonable accommodations for such requests.

Patients may file complaints with their health care providers or directly to the Office of Civil Rights (OCR) of the U.S. Department of Health and Human Services. Providers must give their patients information about where and how to file such complaints.

Impact on Providers

Providers must have written policies and procedures to protect the privacy of their patients' health information. These policies and procedures must describe which employees (and other business associates) may have access to private information and how and when that information may be used and disclosed.

Providers must train their employees on privacy standards and identify one person who is responsible for enforcing policies and procedures. Disciplinary action must be invoked when violations occur.

There are certain, limited circumstances when providers may disclose otherwise private information as part of their "public responsibility." This includes emergency situations, identification of the deceased or cause of death, public health needs, approved research studies, judicial proceedings, some law enforcement situations, and efforts related to security and national defense.

For More Information

The Office of Civil Rights of the U.S. Department of Health and Human Services enforces HIPAA privacy standards. The OCR provides guidance and technical assistance materials to answer questions and ensure compliance. OCR representatives participate in conferences, association meetings, and other forums to provide out-reach and information. Guidance and technical assistance materials are available at http://www.hhs.gov/ocr/hipaa/assist.html. A toll-free information line is available at (866) 627–7748.

The OCR investigates complaints and may impose civil monetary penalties. The U.S. Department of Justice conducts investigations when criminal violations are suspected. Penalties may include fines and prison sentences.

Appendix B

SAMPLE JOB DESCRIPTION

Spruce Family Medicine Clinic
Greentree, IN

Job Title: Certified Medical Assistant
Job Code: B254
Job Family: Clinical
Pay Range: MB7
Status: Non-exempt
Supervisory Responsibility: No
Reports to: Office Manager
Effective Date: January, 2006

SUMMARY

In addition to demonstrating core behaviors and standards of service expected of all employees, incumbent performs routine patient care and administrative procedures to assist physicians and nurses in examining and treating patients in a medical office setting.

ESSENTIAL DUTIES

Essential duties include but are not limited to:

1. Greets patients, answers telephones, schedules appointments
2. Provides care to patients, prepares patients for examinations
3. Assists the physician during the examination
4. Explains treatment procedures to patients
5. Takes medical histories, records vital signs
6. Performs ECGs, removes sutures, changes dressings
7. Instructs patients about medications and special diets
8. Collects laboratory specimens, performs basic laboratory tests
9. Forwards prescriptions to a pharmacy
10. Updates and files patient medical records

---

11. Performs clerical functions and insurance billing
12. Maintains medical equipment and inventory of supplies
13. Maintains a clean, safe, orderly environment

QUALIFICATIONS

Education: Graduation from accredited Medical Assistant program. Proof of high school diploma or GED. Certificate of Completion or Associate of Science Degree in Medical Assisting.

Experience: No experience required. One year relevant work experience preferred.

Certification: Certification by the American Association of Medical Assistants or the American Registry of Medical Assistants required.

KNOWLEDGE/SKILLS/ABILITIES

Incumbent will demonstrate the ability to:
- perform and assist with diagnostic and therapeutic procedures
- conduct medical office procedures and operate medical office equipment
- communicate and document clinical and administrative information
- apply knowledge of sterile technique, infection control, and safety precautions
- apply age specific competencies
- establish and maintain effective working relationships with patients and staff
- demonstrate good customer service and conflict resolution skills
- establish priorities, organize tasks, and manage time efficiently
- allocate and utilize resources cost-effectively
- remain calm in stressful situations
- display effective interpersonal and team skills
- present a professional image as a representative of the practice

Computer skills:
- demonstrate proficiency in Microsoft Word, Excel, Access, and Outlook
- ability to perform clinic-specific computer applications and learn new applications and procedures

Additional qualifications may be required for any particular position. Employees may be expected to perform duties in addition to those presented in this description.

Appendix C

SAMPLE PERFORMANCE EVALUATION

Employee Name _____ Employee Number _____

Job Title/Job Code _____ Department/Unit _____

Supervisor Name _____ Supervisor Title _____

Time period covered by evaluation: From _____ To _____

Date of supervisor meeting with employee (evaluation date) _____

Rating Scale

Evaluate each performance factor using the following 1 to 5 scale:

5   Exceptional, consistently exceeds expectations

4   Highly effective, consistently meets and at times exceeds expectations

3   Effective, consistently meets expectations

2   Needs improvement, occasionally fails to meet expectations

1   Not effective, consistently fails to meet expectations

Part 1: Core Behaviors   Rating

1. Communication Skills   _____
2. Teamwork/Interpersonal Skills   _____
3. Problem Solving Skills   _____
4. Organizational/Time Management Skills   _____
5. Respect for Diversity   _____
6. Service Excellence/Customer Service   _____
7. Support for Quality Improvement   _____
8. Support for Cost Effective Operations   _____
9. Support for Corporate Mission and Values   _____

Comments:

Part 2: Personal Characteristics   <u>Rating</u>

1. Appearance   _____
2. Attitude   _____
3. Initiative   _____
4. Adaptability, flexibility   _____
5. Reliability, trustworthiness   _____
6. Judgment   _____
7. Ethics, integrity   _____
8. Stress management   _____
9. Accountability   _____

Comments:

Part 3: Job-Specific Competencies   <u>Rating</u>

1. Greets patients, answers telephones, schedules appointments   _____
2. Provides care to patients, prepares patients for examinations   _____
3. Assists the physician during the examination   _____
4. Explains treatment procedures to patients   _____
5. Takes medical histories, records vital signs   _____
6. Performs ECGs, removes sutures, changes dressings   _____
7. Instructs patients about medications and special diets   _____
8. Collects laboratory specimens, performs basic laboratory tests   _____
9. Forwards prescriptions to a pharmacy   _____
10. Updates and files patient medical records   _____
11. Performs clerical functions and insurance billing   _____
12. Maintains medical equipment and inventory of supplies   _____
13. Maintains a clean, safe, orderly environment   _____

Comments:

Part 4: Overall Performance

Attendance/punctuality   _____

Technical knowledge   _____

Quality of work   _____

Quantity of work, productivity   _____

Comments:

Part 5: Improvement Plans (if applicable)

Identify improvement plans for each performance factor rated 2 or below:

Comments:

Part 6: Achievements and Recognition

List special achievements, awards, designations, or other types of recognition during this evaluation period:

Comments:

Part 7: Goals and Professional Development Activities

List at least one measurable goal and a self-development activity for the upcoming evaluation period:

Comments:

EMPLOYEE COMMENTS:

_____

_____

_____

SIGNATURES

Employee Signature _____ Date _____
(Signature does not necessarily indicate agreement with evaluation ratings.)

Supervisor Signature_____ Date _____

Approved by: Name _____ Title _____

      Signature _____ Date _____

(Submit completed and signed original to Human Resources; copy given to the employee; copy maintained in the employee's departmental file.)

Appendix D

SAMPLE RÉSUMÉ

Jane Jones, A.S., CMA
123 Maple Street
Greentree, IN 47777
phone: 317/333-4444
email: jjones@mail.net

Objective
Seeking full-time employment as a Certified Medical Assistant with clinical and administrative responsibilities.

Education
Greentree Community College, Greentree, IN
A.S. degree in Medical Assisting, April 3, 2007

Professional Certification
Certified Medical Assistant
American Association of Medical Assistants, April 20, 2007

Experience
Student Extern
Cherry Hill Pediatrics Center, Greentree, IN
December 1, 2006 to January 31, 2007
Poplar Grove Family Practice Center, Poplar Grove, IN
February 3 to March 30, 2007
performed medical assisting clinical and administrative duties

Hospice Unit Volunteer, Greentree Baptist Hospital, Greentree, IN
June 1 to September 31, 2006
answered telephones, delivered flowers, staffed the information desk

Nursing Assistant, Shady Dell Rehab Center, Elm City, IN
January 3 to May 30, 2006
fed and bathed residents, assisted with recreation activities, filed paperwork

Student Photographer, Greentree Gazette, Greentree Community College
March 15, 2007 to present
produce digital photographs, attend editorial meetings, assist graphic artists

Personal
Hobbies: horticulture, photography, antiques
Marital status: single, no children

Appendix E

SAMPLE RÉSUMÉ COVER LETTER

Ms. Jane Jones
123 Maple Street
Greentree, IN 47777

May 20, 2007

Mr. John Johnson
Office Manager
Spruce Family Medicine Clinic
567 Spruce Street
Greentree, IN 47777

Dear Mr. Johnson:

I am writing in response to your ad for a Certified Medical Assistant which appeared in the Greentree Reporter on May 22.

I graduated from the Greentree Community College Medical Assistant Program with an A.S. degree on April 3, 2007, and passed the American Association of Medical Assistants certification examination on April 20. I worked at the Cherry Hill Pediatrics Center in Greentree and the Poplar Grove Family Practice Center in Poplar Grove to complete my externship requirements.

While enrolled as a student at GCC, I spent four months volunteering in the Greentree Baptist Hospital hospice unit and worked part-time for six months as a nursing assistant at the Shady Dell Rehab Center in Elm City. For the past two months I've served as the student photographer for our college's newspaper, the GCC Gazette.

I have enclosed my resume and am available for an interview at your convenience. Please contact me at 333/4444 or jjones@mail.net should you have questions or need additional information. I'm looking forward to meeting you and learning more about employment opportunities with the Spruce Family Medicine Clinic.

Sincerely,

Jane Jones, A.S., CMA
333/4444
jjones@mail.net

Appendix F

SAMPLE JOB APPLICATION FORM

It is our policy to comply with all applicable state and federal laws prohibiting discrimination in employment on race, age, color, sex, religion, national origin or other protected classification.

Instructions: Print clearly in black or blue ink. Answer all questions. Sign and date the form.

PERSONAL INFORMATION

First Name   _____

Middle Name   _____

Last Name   _____

SS Number   _____

Street Address   _____

     _____

City, State, Zip Code _____

Telephone Number   (_____) _____

Are you over 18 years old?   Yes _____ No _____

Are you a U.S. citizen or otherwise authorized to work in the U.S. on an unrestricted basis?

Yes _____ No _____

Have you ever been convicted of, or pleaded no contest to, a felony?

(Conviction will not necessarily disqualify an applicant for employment.)

Yes_____ No_____

If yes, describe conditions:_____

POSITION and AVAILABILITY

Position Applied For _____

Are there any hours, shifts or days you cannot or will not work?

No _____ Yes: _____

Preferences:

Status Part-time _____ Full-time_____ Supplemental _____

Shift Day _____ Evening _____ Night _____ Weekends _____

Are you available to work overtime as required? Yes _____ No _____

What date are you available to start work? _____

EDUCATION

High School/GED Education:

Have you earned a high school diploma or GED? Yes _____ No _____

Awarded by _____

Date awarded _____

Postsecondary Education (List all schools attended; use a separate sheet of paper if necessary)

School Name _____

School Address _____

_____

Field of Study _____

Degree/Diploma _____

Graduation Date _____

Other Postsecondary Education:

School Name _____

School Address _____

_____

Field of Study _____

Degree/Diploma _____

Graduation Date _____

Professional License/Certification/Registration:

Title/Date _____

Awarded by _____

Expiration date _____

Other Training and Skills:

_____

_____

_____

Awards/Recognition:

_____

_____

EMPLOYMENT HISTORY

(List all employment during the past five years; use a separate sheet of paper if necessary)

Present or Last Position:

Employer: _____

Address: _____

_____

Supervisor:

Name _____

Title _____

Phone _____

Email _____

Your Position:

Job Title _____

Employment dates From:_____ To: _____

Responsibilities _____

Reason for leaving _____

Previous Position:

Employer: _____

Address: _____

_____

Supervisor:

Name _____

Title _____

Phone _____

Email _____

Your Position:

Job Title _____

Employment dates From: _____ To: _____

Responsibilities _____

Reason for leaving _____

May We Contact Your Present Employer?

Yes _____ No _____

How did you learn of this opening? _____

Have you ever worked here before? No _____ Yes _____

If yes, dates of employment: From _____ To _____

Job title _____

References:

1) Name _____ Title _____

   Address _____ Phone _____

   Relationship to you _____

2) Name _____ Title _____

   Address _____ Phone _____

   Relationship to you _____

3) Name _____ Title _____

   Address _____ Phone _____

   Relationship to you _____

I certify that information contained in this application is true and complete.

I understand that false information may be grounds for not hiring me or for immediate termination of employment at any point in the future if I am hired.

I authorize the verification of any or all information listed above.

Printed Name _____

Signature _____

Date Signed _____

Appendix G

SAMPLE INTERVIEW FOLLOW-UP LETTER

Ms. Jane Jones
123 Maple Street
Greentree, IN 47777

June 10, 2007

Mr. John Johnson
Office Manager
Spruce Family Medicine Clinic
567 Spruce Street
Greentree, IN 47777

Dear Mr. Johnson:

Thank you for the opportunity to interview with you and Dr. Seymour yesterday for a CMA position. Having met you and your colleagues and toured the facility, I am very excited about the prospect of joining the Spruce Family Medicine team.

As promised, here is the contact information for my three references:

1)   Mary Woods, RN, CMA, Director, CGG Medical Assisting Program
            phone: 317/333-5555; email: mwoods@gcc.edu
2)   Laura Allen, RN, Hospice Unit Manager, Greentree Baptist Hospital
            phone 317/333-6666; email lallen@gbh.org
3)   Martin Moser, MD, Chief Medical Officer, Cherry Hill Pediatrics Center
            phone 317/333-7777; email mmoser@chpc.com

I believe that my education, experience, and commitment to quality care and service excellence make me well qualified for the CMA position.

Thank you again for the interview and I look forward to hearing from you soon.

Sincerely,

Jane Jones, A.S., CMA
333-4444
jjones@mail.net

Index